Narjes ABID
Asma ZGOLLI
Khaled BOUZAIDI

Massive hemoptysis: place of pre-embolization bronchial angioscanq

Narjes ABID
Asma ZGOLLI
Khaled BOUZAIDI

Massive hemoptysis: place of pre-embolization bronchial angioscanq

ScienciaScripts

Imprint
Any brand names and product names mentioned in this book are subject to trademark, brand or patent protection and are trademarks or registered trademarks of their respective holders. The use of brand names, product names, common names, trade names, product descriptions etc. even without a particular marking in this work is in no way to be construed to mean that such names may be regarded as unrestricted in respect of trademark and brand protection legislation and could thus be used by anyone.

Cover image: www.ingimage.com

This book is a translation from the original published under ISBN 978-620-6-72315-8.

Publisher:
Sciencia Scripts
is a trademark of
Dodo Books Indian Ocean Ltd. and OmniScriptum S.R.L publishing group

120 High Road, East Finchley, London, N2 9ED, United Kingdom
Str. Armeneasca 28/1, office 1, Chisinau MD-2012, Republic of Moldova, Europe
Printed at: see last page
ISBN: 978-620-8-24295-4

Signing sessions

I dedicate this work

To my parents Ibtissem and Sabeur,

For your support, your unconditional love and your patience.

For everything you've done for me along the way.

It's for you and thanks to your sacrifices and dedication that I'm becoming a doctor.

Thank you for everything. I can't express how grateful and thankful I am to you.

I love you with all my heart.

To my little sister Mariem,

For our complicity and our union.

For the joy that your presence brings me in my life.

For your love, your patience and your efforts.

Thank you so much.

In memory of my grandfathers Baba Zgolli and Baba Taher and Mima,

For showering me with love since I was born. You are always present in my heart. May God welcome you into his Paradise.

To my grandmother Nabiha

For your encouragement and your love. May God keep you for us.

To my dearest *Senda, Sameh, Maryem Chetoui, Rania, Houssem, Yosr, Mariem Gouiaa, Salim, Oussama, Mohamed, Wejdene and Achref.*

For the love and happiness you give me every day.

Nothing can express the love and esteem I have for you.

Please find in this work the testimony of my great love and respect.

To my aunts and uncles and cousins

Thank you for your encouragement, and I wish you every happiness and prosperity.

Acknowledgements

To our teacher and chairman of the thesis jury,
Professor SaoussenHantous-Zannad
Head of Medical Imaging Department, Abdelrahmen Mami Hospital, Ariana

You do us an immense honour by chairing this jury. I was lucky enough to be your student and to benefit from your scientific and human expertise. I hope that I will have the opportunity to refine my knowledge through a period of specialisation in your department. Please accept the expression of my deepest respect and thanks.

To our master and thesis judge,
Professor Leila Charrada-Ben Farhat
Head of Medical Imaging Department, Mongi Slim Hospital La Marsa

You have done me a great honour by agreeing to judge this thesis. You taught me the basics of radiology and thanks to you I have become passionate about it. I have learnt from your scientific and human qualities and from your dedication. May this work bear witness to my deep gratitude.

To our master and thesis judge,
Professor HediaGhrairi
Head of Medical Imaging Department, Mohamed Taher Maamouri Hospital, Nabeul

Thank you for doing me the honour of agreeing to sit on the jury for this thesis. Thank you for your warm welcome and kindness. Please find here the expression of my most sincere considerations.

To our master and thesis judge,
Professor Myriam Jrad
Head of Medical Imaging Department, Hôpital Charles Nicolle Tunis

You have done me a great honour by agreeing to judge this thesis. You have made a major contribution to my training. I was lucky enough to be your student for the whole of my third year and I was able to benefit from your experience and your rigorous approach to my work. Please accept the expression of my great gratitude.

To our teacher and thesis rapporteur,
Professor Besma Dhahri Ourari
Head of Pneumology Department, Hôpital La Rabta Tunis

Thank you for your availability, your warm and smiling welcome and your understanding. Please accept my highest esteem and respectful consideration.

To our master and thesis supervisor,
Professor Khaled Bouzaidi
Head of Medical Imaging Department, Mohamed Taher Maamouri Hospital, Nabeul

You agreed to supervise and support me during the preparation of this thesis. I would like to thank you for your patience, your constant availability and your unfailing kindness and help. I am delighted and grateful to have had the chance to work with you and benefit from your scientific support. Please accept my sincere gratitude and deepest respect.

To our teacher and thesis co-director,
Doctor Narjes Abid
Pneumology Department, Mohamed Taher Maamouri Hospital, Nabeul

I'd like to thank you very much for the quality of your guidance, your tireless availability and your help. It has been a pleasure to work with you. Please find here, dear master, the expression of my deepest considerations and my great gratitude.

To our master
Dr Tibaoui Ahmed
Medical Imaging Department, Salhoul Hospital, Sousse

I would like to thank you very much for all your help, your warm welcome and your availability. It was a pleasure working with you. Please accept my deepest sympathy and gratitude.

TABLE OF CONTENTS

INTRODUCTION

Haemoptysis is the release of blood from the subglottic airways during a coughing effort. [1,2]. The severity of haemoptysis depends on its size and recurrence.

Low-intensity haemoptysis is defined as the emission of less than 50 cc of blood / 24 hours and requires an aetiological investigation as it represents an alarming sign of multiple pathologies.

Severe haemoptysis is defined as the emission of more than 200 cc of bright red blood in one or more episodes per 24 hours, often requiring emergency bronchial embolisation. Haemoptysis is considered massive when the quantity of blood emitted exceeds 300 cc / 24 hours [3-5]. This is a rare but serious form of haemoptysis, which can be life-threatening, with a high mortality rate estimated at between 30% and 50%. [6,7]. The patient dies of asphyxia in the absence of urgent and adequate treatment. [8]. To date, there is no consensus on the best therapeutic approach, based on clinical data and, above all, on additional investigations such as chest X-ray, bronchoscopy, thoracic angioscan and conventional angiography, which is systematically performed before the embolisation procedure.

The main aim of this paraclinical investigation is to identify the precise site of the bleed and the aetiology of the haemoptysis in order to guide percutaneous and medical and/or surgical treatment of the causative pathology respectively. Whether thoracic angioscanning should be performed prior to bronchial embolisation remains debatable. Few previous studies, especially in Africa and particularly in Tunisia, have considered its contribution to determining the site of bleeding for catheterisation directed at the artery to be embolised and to assessing the prognosis of patients after bronchial artery embolisation.

For this reason, we carried out a cross-sectional study including 58 radio-clinical observations of patients hospitalised for massive haemoptysis, investigated by thoracic CT angiography and angiography before bronchial embolisation.

The objectives were to

- To describe the role of thoracic CT angiography in determining the site of bleeding in massive haemoptysis, comparing its data with that of conventional pre-embolisation angiography.
- Look for radiological severity criteria predictive of recurrence or mortality.

METHODS

1. Type and location of study

Descriptive study with cross-sectional collection of data from 58 patients, 41 of whom were hospitalised in the Pneumology Department of the Mohamed Taher Maâmouri University Hospital in Nabeul for the management of massive haemoptysis, investigated by thoracic DTA in the Medical Imaging Department of the same hospital and 17 other patients investigated in the Medical Imaging Department of the Sahloul Hospital in Sousse. All patients were treated by bronchial embolisation at Sahloul Hospital, Sousse, and the study lasted 13 years and 5 months, from June 2008 to November 2021.

2. P atients

2.1. Inclusion criteria

Patients were included in the study:

- ✓ presenting with massive haemoptysis due to its initial abundance or its recurrence during hospitalisation despite well-managed medical treatment.
- ✓ explored by a thoracic CT scan.
- ✓ who had undergone angiography followed by bronchial artery embolisation.

2.2. Non-inclusion criteria

Patients not included in the study were :

- ✓ with haemoptysis initially considered severe but controlled by medical treatment alone and not requiring treatment by bronchial artery embolisation.
- ✓ with an absolute contraindication to EAB.
- ✓ with missing imaging (missing CDs or CT scans).
- ✓ with missing data from angiography.

3. M ethodes

3.1. Data collection

The main source of data was the patients' medical records. These data were transmitted on an analytical form (Appendix 1) containing the following data:

3.1.1. Clinical and epidemiological data

- ✓ The patient's identity.
- ✓ Age.

- ✓ Sex.
- ✓ A history of cardiovascular and respiratory diseases (in particular tuberculosis and bronchial dilatation) and pulmonary neoplasia.
- ✓ The concept of smoking.
- ✓ General and functional clinical signs, specifying whether or not respiratory distress was present on admission.

3.1.2. Biological data

- ✓ Blood count (CBC).
- ✓ Haemostasis test.

3.1.3. Data from bronchial fibroscopy

Depending on the initial clinical presentation, patients were investigated by bronchial fibroscopy performed by a senior respirologist using an optical fiberscope with video column. The following parameters were studied

- ✓ The condition and mobility of the vocal cords.
- ✓ Freedom of the trachea.
- ✓ Macroscopic appearance of the bronchi :
  - Normal, inflammatory or hyper-vascularised.
  - Reduction or increase in bronchial calibre.
  - The presence or absence of extrinsic distortion, infiltration or compression.
- ✓ The presence of bleeding and its location: right or left bronchial tree or bilateral.

3.1.4. Radiological data

3.1.4.1. Chest X-ray

The semiological elements studied were :

- **Signs associated with bleeding**
  - ✓ An alveolar syndrome diagnosed when :
    - Nodular opacities with blurred, ill-defined contours, sometimes confluent.
    - Systematic, segmental or lobar opacities with an aerated bronchogram.
  - ✓ Interstitial syndrome, identified by :

- Well-limited parenchymal nodules.
- Interstitial oedema with linear opacities or Kerley A or B lines.
- Reticulo-nodular opacities.
- Blurring of vascular contours in the hilum and peribronchovascular opacities.

o **Signs related to the aetiology of the bleeding**

✓ Excavated opacity.

✓ A well-limited single or multiple opacity.

✓ A poorly defined opacity with a spiculated outline.

✓ Mediastinal adenomegalia.

3.1.4.2. Chest scan

The time taken to perform DMFTs was between 24 and 72 hours after admission.

3.1.4.2.1. Technical

The CT examinations were carried out using a 16-detector scanner made by *GENERAL ELECTRIC HEALTHCARE*, which came into service in 2012 in the Medical Imaging Department of the Mohamed Taher Maâmouri University Hospital in Nabeul, or a 16-detector scanner made by the same manufacturer, which came into service in 2004 at the Sahloul Hospital.

A cranio-caudal helical volume acquisition extended from the base of the neck to the upper pole of the right kidney in deep inspiration followed by apnoea maintained for approximately 15 seconds.

The origin of the supra-aortic trunks and diaphragmatic arteries was included in order to search for the origin of any non-bronchial systemic arteries that should be identified prior to bronchial artery embolisation (BAE).

Acquisition was performed immediately after injection of non-ionic iodinated contrast medium (ICP) concentrated at 350 or 370 mg/dl. The aim was to opacify both the bronchial and pulmonary arteries.

An injection-free acquisition of PDCI, centred on the adrenals, was performed whenever pulmonary neoplasia was suspected.

The precautions taken were :

- The search for a possible hypersensitivity reaction to PDCI.

- Checking renal function by calculating creatinine clearance.
- Verification of the presence of a good calibre 18 Gauge venous line at the level of the permeable elbow.
- The flow rate was 3.5 to 4 ml/s.
- The quantity of PDCI was calculated as a function of acquisition time, flow rate and kilovoltage. The quality criterion was vascular enhancement greater than 300 Hounsfield Units. The region of interest (ROI) was positioned on the descending aorta.
- The scanner parameters (kilovoltages and milliamperes) have been adapted to the patient's weight to obtain the best image quality with the lowest possible radiation exposure.

The reconstructions were carried out using a section thickness of 1.25 mm and an interval of 1 mm with high-resolution lung and soft tissue filters.

3.1.4.2.2. Interpretation

The scanner data was transferred to dedicated post-processing consoles (Advantage 4.6). The scans were read by two radiologists, one junior and one senior, using multiplanar reconstructions and post-processing software such as MIP (Maximum Intensity Projection) or minIP (Minimum Intensity Projection).

Readings were taken from different windows: mediastinal, pulmonary and bone.

3.1.4.2.2.1. Basic thoracic CT semiology

a. Positive diagnosis, topography and extent

Signs pointing to the site of bleeding were specified by looking for [9,10]in the form of :

✓ <u>Ranges of ground-glass hyperdensity [11]</u>

Vertrepoli" represents an increase in the density of the lung parenchyma. The vessels within it remain visible and of normal calibre.

✓ <u>Parenchymal condensations[11]</u>

Parenchymal condensation corresponds to an increase in lung density that blurs the contours of the vessels, unlike "ground-glass" hyperdensities.

✓ <u>Centrilobular micronodules</u>

A micronodule is a focal increase in the density of the lung parenchyma, round in shape with clear, regular or irregular or blurred boundaries and a major axis of less than 3mm.

Centrilobular micronodules are due to a bronchogenic distribution. They are located in the centre of the secondary pulmonary lobules, in contact with the bronchioles and terminal arterioles, far from the pleural interstitium, the peribronchovascular connective sheaths and the interlobular septa.

✓ Regular thickening of the intra- and inter-lobular septa

Defined by abnormal visibility of a thickened intra- or interlobular septum.

✓ Crazy paving" appearance

Defined by regular thickening of the inter- and intra-lobular septa within "ground glass" hyperdensities.

The extent of stigmata of recent bleeding and their topography according to bronchial segmentation were studied.

We have chosen to assess the extent of the disease as a percentage of the number of lung segments affected out of the 20 lung segments:

- Absent: No segment has been reached.
- Moderate: 1 to 25% (1 to 5 segments).
- Range: 25% to 50% (from 6 to 10 segments).
- Severe: 50 to 75% (11 to 15 segments).
- Critical: 75 to 100% (from 16 to 20 segments).

b. Aetiological diagnosis

- Parenchymal abnormalities pointing to the etiology of the bleeding were noted:
  - ✓ Nodule:a nodule is a focal increase in the density of the lung parenchyma, rounded in shape with an average diameter strictly greater than 3mm and less than 30mm.
  - ✓ Mass: corresponds to the same definition of a nodule but with an average diameter greater than 30mm. Its contours may be regular, irregular or spiculated.
  - ✓ Parenchymal condensation: corresponds to an increase in the density of the lung parenchyma, blurring the vascular boundaries. It may be excavated, with cavitation of aerial density, suggestive of tuberculosis.

- ✓ Sequelae of tuberculosis: calcified nodules, retractile condensations, pleural plaques or bronchiectasis.
- ✓ Bronchial dilatation (BDD): defined by an abnormal increase in bronchial caliber with a minor axis greater than the caliber of the adjacent artery or by the absence of a decrease in the caliber of the bronchus over at least 2 cm or by the visibility of the bronchus sub pleural. [12].
- ✓ Signs of parenchymal fibrosis with
  - Honeycomb" images corresponding to regular cystic lesions in strata.
  - Scissural distortion: loss of the regularity of a scissure.
  - Bronchovascular distortion and traction bronchiectasis, with deformation of the bronchial and vascular routes as a result of retraction and a reduction in lung volume.

c. Study of pulmonary vascularisation

- Bronchial and non-bronchial systemic circulation
  - ✓ Bronchial arteries have been defined:
    - Right broncho-intercostal trunk.
    - Right-left common bronchial trunk.
    - Right or left bronchial trunk.
    - Other variants.
  - ✓ A count of pathological bronchial systemic arteries (BSAs) and non-bronchial systemic arteries (NBSAs) traceable on CT was carried out.
  - ✓ For each bronchial artery considered to be responsible for the bleeding, the following information was provided:
    - Its ostium if seen. It is :
      - Orthotopic bronchial systemic if arising from the aorta between D5 and D6[11].
      - Systemic bronchial ectopywhen it arises from the aorta but not opposite D5 and D6, or from the internal mammary artery, subclavian artery, diaphragmatic artery, brachiocephalic or thyro-cervical trunk [11,13,14]. In all cases, these arteries follow the bronchial tubes.

- Non-systemic bronchial when its course is pleural with an opposite thickening exceeding 3mm [11,15]. They enter the thorax outside the pulmonary hilum and do not follow the path of the bronchi.

- Its diameter: at the level of the bronchial bifurcation in the mediastinum. A bronchial artery was considered dilated when its diameter exceeded 2mm.
- Its route through the mediastinum, hilum and/or lung parenchyma.
- Its degree of tortuosity: minimal, moderate or significant.

An artery was considered to be responsible for the bleeding if it was dilated and tortuous.

ATDM was considered capable of detecting an artery responsible for bleeding when it detected its ostium and was able to follow it into the mediastinum.

We looked for dangerous arterial anastomoses, in particular the presence of an anterior spinal artery.

- Pulmonary arterial circulation

  The presence of :

  - ✓ Pulmonary artery embolism.
  - ✓ A pulmonary artery aneurysm.
  - ✓ An arterio-bronchial fistula.

3.1.4.3. Arterial angiography

All patients underwent arterial angiography for EAB.

- A contraindication to this procedure, such as the presence of an anterior spinal artery, was systematically sought. This artery normally arises from the 2ème , 3ème or 4ème right and left intercostal arteries [1,16]. These intercostal arteries may arise from the broncho-intercostal trunk. In these cases, EAB may be complicated by bone marrow ischaemia.
- Patient consent was sought prior to angiography and EAB.
- The aim of EAB was to reduce the blood pressure of pathological vessels weakened by the chronic inflammatory process and to prevent the recruitment of non-bronchial collateral vessels. [17].
- **Production techniques**

1. Patient monitoring with heart rate, blood pressure, electrocardiogram and arterial oxygen saturation.[18].
2. Local anaesthesia with lidocaine at the puncture site.
3. Femoral arterial approach using a 5French stent.
4. Selective catheterisation of bronchial and non-bronchial arteries considered pathological on CTAT using a catheter.
5. Injection of contrast medium.
6. Acquisition of angiographic images.
7. Embolisation of the culprit artery is performed whenever possible.

- The items noted were :
    - The topography of the bleed.
    - Type of bleeding artery: ASB or ASNB.
    - The presence or absence of a parenchymal blush, which corresponds to the passage of CIDP into the lung parenchyma.
    - The presence of a systemic-pulmonary countercurrent shunt in relation to systemic hypervascularisation.
    - The procedure performed, specifying the type of molecules used .
    - The result:
        - Immediate EAB success: defined as immediate cessation of bleeding.
        - Otherwise, embolisation fails.
    - The occurrence of a post-EAB complication: spinal cord ischaemia, cerebellar ischaemia, acute coronary syndrome or bronchial necrosis.

3.1.5. Clinical follow-up data

We defined the duration of follow-up as the period between the date of embolisation and the date of the last consultation, death or end of study.

We defined recurrence as the reappearance of haemoptysis (as assessed by a doctor) regardless of its size. Depending on the time of onset, we considered recurrence :

- Immediate or short-term if it occurs within 03 months of EAB.
- Medium-term if it occurs between 03 months and 1 year after EAB.

- Long-term if it occurs after 01 year.

4. Statistical analysis

Statistical analysis of the data was carried out using IBM SPSS statistics software (Statistical Package for the Social Sciences) version 20.0.

4.1. Statistical tests

Descriptive study

Qualitative variables were described in terms of observed numbers and frequencies (%).

For quantitative variables, the distribution of the data was studied using skewness and kurtosis coefficients and normality tests. These variables were described by means and standard deviation in the case of a normal distribution, and by medians and interquartile ranges in the opposite case.

Analytical study

To analyse the association between two categorical variables, Pearson's chi2 test was used to compare two frequencies if the conditions of application were met, and Fischer's test if they were not.

To analyse the association between a qualitative and a quantitative variable, the non-parametric Mann Whitney test was used.

McNemar's paired tests were used to compare two paired frequencies if the application conditions were met, and Fischer's test was used if they were not.

In the multivariate study, the risk was calculated using the Odds Ratio (OR) with a confidence interval of 95% (IC $)._{95\%}$

To estimate performance, the parameters of sensitivity, specificity, positive predictive value (PPV) and negative predictive value (NPV) were used.

The significance threshold was set at $p \leq 5\%$.

5. Bibliographic research

The bibliography was compiled using Zotero software.

The data for our study were retrieved from :

- PubMed (http://www.ncbi.nlm.nih.gov/pubmed).
- Science direct (http ://www.sciencedirect.com).

- Google Scholar (https://scholar.google.com).
- Elsevier Masson Consulte (https://www.em-consulte.com).

The keywords used were :

- Haemoptysis.
- Angioscanner.
- Angiography.
- Diagnosis.
- Prognosis.
- Balloon catheter embolisation.

6. Ethics and conflicts of interest

Given the retrospective nature of the study, no consent was sought.

Data was collected in such a way as to respect patients' anonymity and the confidentiality of their information.

We have no conflicts of interest to declare in this study.

RESULTS

1. Descriptive study

Fifty-eight patients were included in the study.

1.1. Characteristics of the population

1.1.1. Age

The average age of patients was 55.3. The age groups most affected were 40-59 and 60-79(Figure 1).

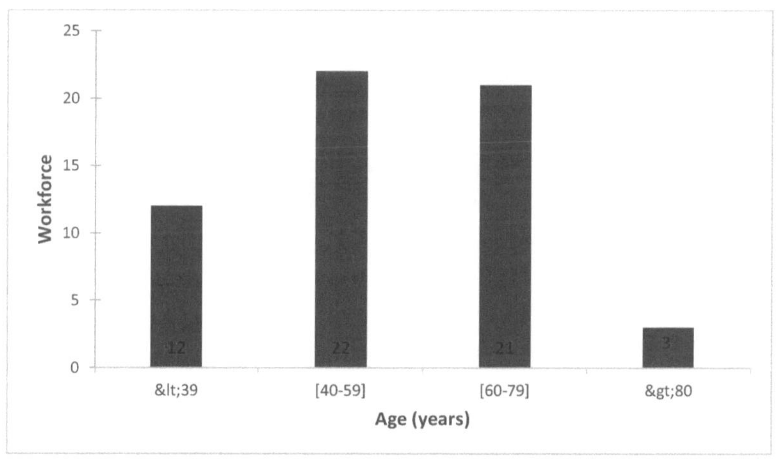

Figure 1 Breakdown of patients by age group.

1.1.2. Gender

The male/female sex ratio was 2.8 (Figure2).

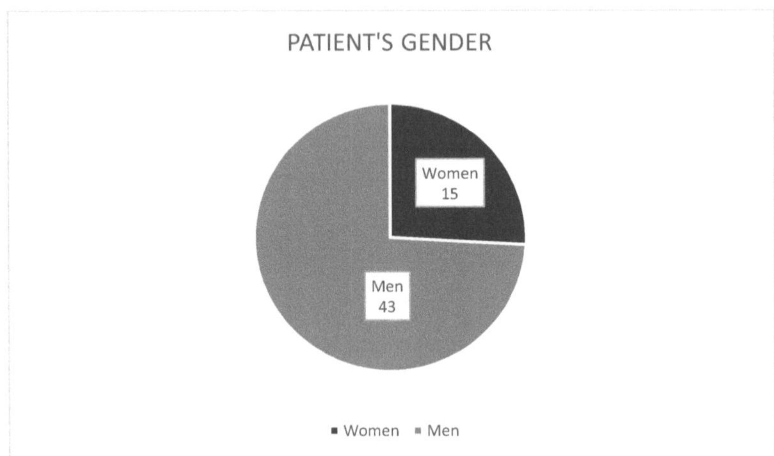

Figure2 Breakdown of patients by sex .

1.1.3. Habits

1.1.3.1. Smoking

Approximately two-thirds of patients were smokers (Figure3).

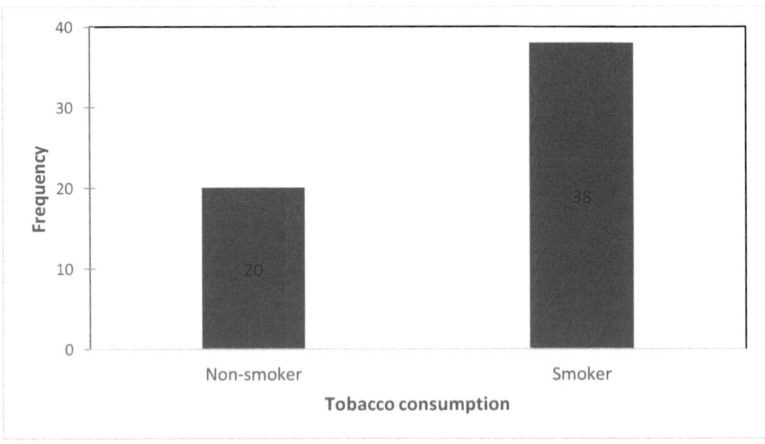

Figure3 Distribution of patients according to smoking habits.

1.1.4. Pathological history

1.1.4.1. Cardiovascular diseases

Seventeen patients had a history of cardiovascular disease. These histories are summarised in Table I.

Table I Breakdown of patients by history of cardiovascular disease

Cardiovascular history	N (%)
Hypertension	14 (24,1%)
Heart disease	5 (8,6%)

1.1.4.2. Respiratory diseases

Fourteen patients (24.1%) had a known history of respiratory disease at the time of the study (table II).

Table II Distribution of patients according to history of respiratory disease

Respiratory history	N (%)
Bronchial dilatation	8 (13,8%)
Pulmonary tuberculosis	4 (6,9%)
Known lung neoplasia	2 (3,4%)

1.2. Clinical study

1.2.1. Respiratory signs

1.2.1.1. Haemoptysis

All the patients included in the study presented with haemoptysis judged to be massive.

1.2.1.2. Severe acute respiratory distress

Two out of 58 patients presented with acute respiratory distress on admission and required resuscitation before being transferred to the respiratory department.

1.2.1.3. Oxygen saturation

Finger pulse oxygen saturation was recorded for all patients on admission, enabling them to be divided into four categories(Figure4).

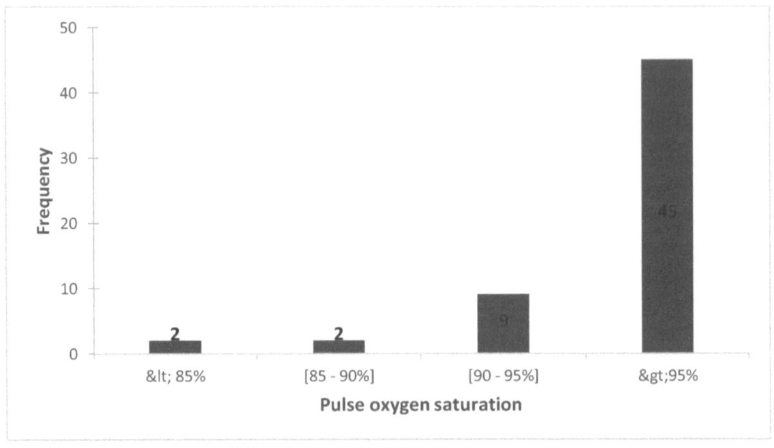

Figure4 Distribution of patients according to pulse oxygen saturation on admission .

1.2.1.4. Respiratory frequency

The minimum respiratory rate was 14 cpm (cycles per minute) and the maximum was 20 cpm, with an average of 15.8 cpm.

1.2.2. Extra-respiratory signs

Five patients presented extra-respiratory signs as detailed in Table III.

Table III Extra-respiratory signs

Extra-respiratory signs	N (%)
Neurological signs	03 (5,2%)
Peripheral adenopathy	01 (1,7%)
State of shock	01 (1,7%)

1.2.3. Percutaneous treatment by bronchial artery embolisation

All patients included in the study underwent EAB at different times.

1.2.4. Time between onset of symptoms and bronchial artery embolisation

The average time between haemoptysis and embolisation was 10.3 days, with a minimum of 1.5 days and a maximum of 74 days.

1.2.5. Time between positive diagnosis and bronchial artery embolisation

The average time between diagnosis and percutaneous treatment with EAB was 5.4 days, with extremes of 0 days and 21 days.

1.2.6. Length of hospital stay

The average length of hospitalisation in the pneumology department was 11.8 days, with extremes of 03 days and 60 days.

1.2.6.1. Length of hospital stay before embolisation

The average was 6 days, with a minimum of 0 days and a maximum of 39 days.

1.2.6.2. Length of hospitalisation after embolisation

The average was 5.5 days, with a minimum of 01 days and a maximum of 21 days.

1.3. Endoscopic data

Of the 58 patients included in the study, 51 (88%) underwent bronchial fibroscopy prior to percutaneous treatment with EAB. Bronchial fibroscopy was performed remotely for the remaining 07 patients (12%) and repeated remotely for a further 11 patients.

1.3.1. Endoscopy conditions

Exploration was complete in 36 patients, i.e. in 62.1% of cases. It was incomplete in 24.1% of cases because of impassable bronchial stenosis or obstruction, or major bleeding.

The procedure was stopped in 8 cases (13.8%) because of poor tolerance.

1.3.2. Results of bronchial endoscopy

In cases investigated prior to EAB, bronchial fibroscopy was normal in 11 patients (21.5% of cases) and pathological in 40 cases (78.4% of patients investigated) (Table IV).

Table IV Distribution of patients according to the site of bleeding at endoscopy

Site of bleeding		N (%)
Undetermined		15 (29,4%)
Known	Right bronchial tree	21 (41,1%)
	Left bronchial tree	15 (29,4%)

1.4. Imaging data

1.4.1. Chest X-ray

A chest X-ray was performed in all cases. It was normal in 31% of patients (n=18) and pathological in the remainder.

1.4.1.1. Results related to the site of bleeding

Twenty-four patients had radiographic signs suggesting the site of bleeding (Table V).

Table V Distribution of patients according to radiographic signs pointing to the site of bleeding

Radiographic abnormality		N (%)
No		34 (58,7%)
Interstitial syndrome		6 (10,3%)
Alveolar syndrome	Unilateral	15 (25,9%)
	Bilateral	3 (5,2%)

1.4.1.2. Results related to the etiology of the bleeding

Thirty-seven patients had chest X-ray findings suggesting the aetiology of the bleeding (Table VI).

Table VI Distribution of patients according to radiographic signs suggesting the aetiology of bleeding

Radiographic abnormality			N (%)
Nodule			4 (6,9%)
Micronodules			4 (6,9%)
Atelectasis			1 (1,7%)
Opacity	Round	Proximal	8 (13,8%)
		Peripheral	1 (1,7%)
	Spiculated	Proximal	7 (12,1%)
		Peripheral	0 (0%)
Excavation			4 (6,9%)

1.4.2. Thoracic CT angiography

All patients underwent a thoracic CT scan. CT scans were normal in 4 patients (6.9% of cases) and pathological in all other cases.

1.4.2.1. Signs pointing to the site of bleeding

1.4.2.1.1. Frequency

Stigmata of recent bleeding were found in 46 cases, i.e. 79.3% of scans (Figure5).

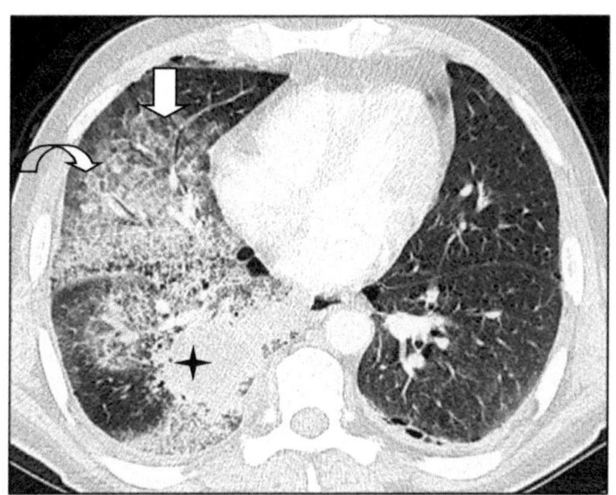

Figure5 Axial section of a thoracic CT angiogram in a patient presenting with massive haemoptysis showingtigmata of recent bleeding in the right lung with areas of "ground-glass" hyperdensity (arrow), parenchymal condensation (star) and a "crazy paving" appearance (curved arrow).

1.4.2.1.2. Scope

The mean number of lung segments affected was 6.6, with extremes of 1 and 19 (Table VII).

Table VII Distribution of patients according to the extent of bleeding stigmata at ATDM

Extent of stigmata of recent bleeding	N (%)
Absent	12 (20,7%)
Moderate **1-25% (1 to 5 segments)**	19(32,8%)
Scope **26-50% (6 to 10 segments)**	14(24,1%)

Severe **51-75% (6 to 15 segments)**	8 (13,8%)
Review **76-100% (16 to 20 segments)**	5 (8,6%)

1.4.2.1.3. Predominantly

For each scan, the main site of bleeding was noted (Table VIII) except in 3 cases where the stigmata of recent bleeding were diffuse and bilateral.

Table VIII Distribution of patients according to the predominance of bleeding stigmata at ATDM

Location	Frequency N(%)
A right lobe	20 (34,5%)
A left lobe (Figure6)	15 (25,9%)
A right lobe and a left lobe	2 (3,4%)
Right lung	4 (6,9%)
Left lung	2 (3,4%)

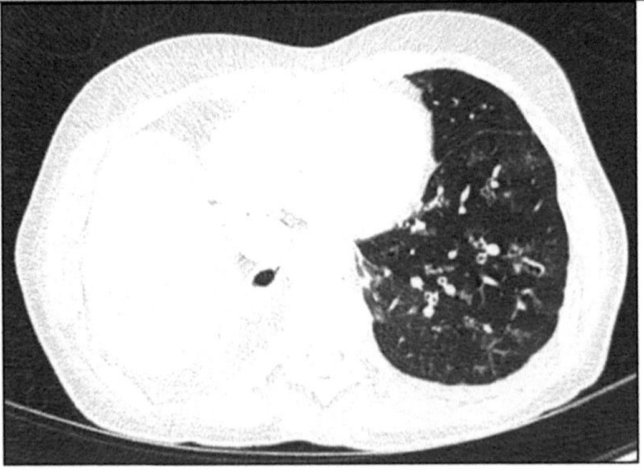

Figure6 Axial section of a thoracic CT angiogram in the parenchymal window showing bleeding stigmata centred in the left lower lobe in the form of a few ground-glass areas associated with DDB.

1.4.2.2. Frequency of parenchymal and mediastinal signs suggesting the aetiology of massive haemoptysis

After reviewing the 58 thoracic CT scans, we have summarised the results in Table IX.

Table IX Frequency of scans suggesting the aetiology of massive haemoptysis

Scannographic sign	Frequency N (%)
Parenchymal nodule	10 (17,2%)
Suspicious mass	13 (22,4%)
Tuberculous cave (Figure7)	7 (12,1%)
Sequelae of pulmonary tuberculosis	8 (13,8%)
Pulmonary fibrosis	4 (6,8%)
Non-systematic parenchymal condensation	3 (5,2%)
Bronchial dilatation(Figure8)	30 (51,7%)
Parenchymal collapse	8 (13,8%)

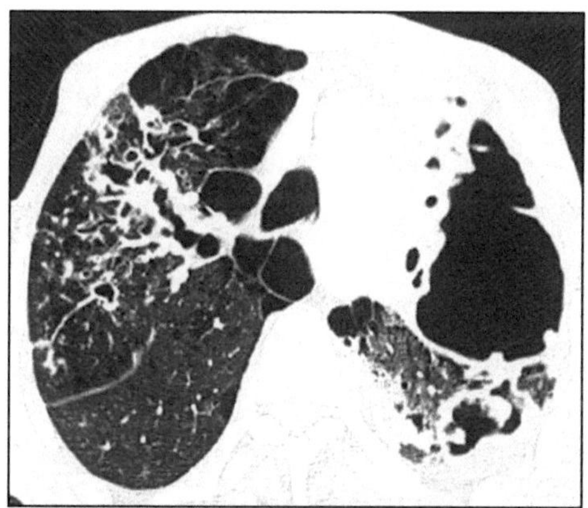

Figure7 Axial section of a CT angiogram in the parenchymal window showing parenchymal condensation in the left upper lobe with cavities consistent with the sequelae of tuberculosis.

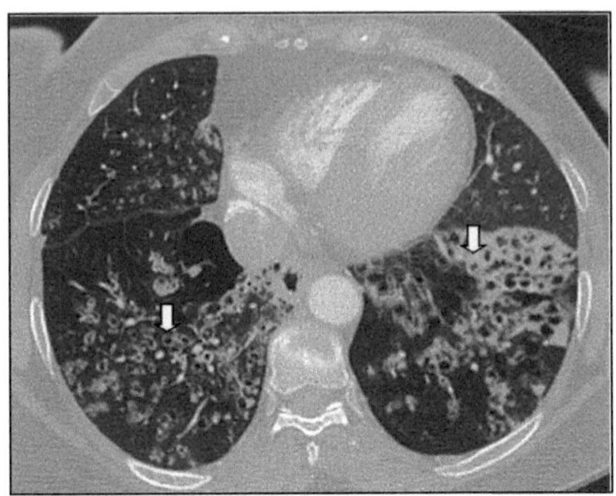

Figure8 Axial section of a thoracic CT angiogram in the parenchymal window showing bilateral foci of DDB (arrows) associated with diffuse bronchial parietal thickening and parenchymal condensation.

1.4.2.3. Etiology retained on thoracic CT scan

At the end of the clinico-biological study and after analysis of the DTAs, a final aetiology for the bleeding was chosen for each patient (Table X).

Table X Etiologies of bleeding detected by CT angiography

Etiology	Frequency N(%)
1. Infectious :	
a. Tuberculosis	4 (6,9%)
b. Aspergilloma (Figure9)	2 (3,4%)
2. Tumour :	
a. Bronchopulmonary cancer	11 (19,0%)
b. Lung metastases	2 (3,4%)
3. Bronchiectasis :	22 (37,9%)
4. Associations :	
a. Tuberculosis and bronchopulmonary cancer:	1 (1,7%)
b. Bronchopulmonary cancer and bronchiectasis:	1 (1,7%)
c. Tuberculosis and bronchiectasis:	1 (1,7%)
5. Pneumoconiosis complicated by fibrosis :	1 (1,7%)
6. Pulmonary and vascular malformations :	
a. Abnormal venous return with secondary pulmonary hypertension:	1 (1,7%) 1 (1,7%)
b. Bronchial arterial fistula :	1 (1,7%)

c. Pulmonary artery aneurysm :	1 (1,7%)
d. Pulmonary sequestration :	
7. Idiopathic :	9 (15,5%)

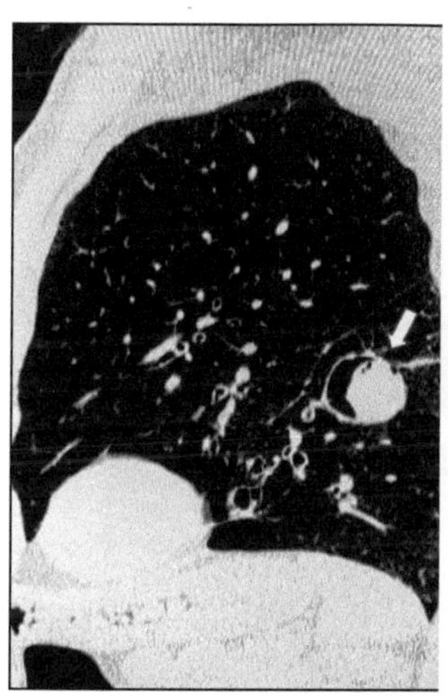
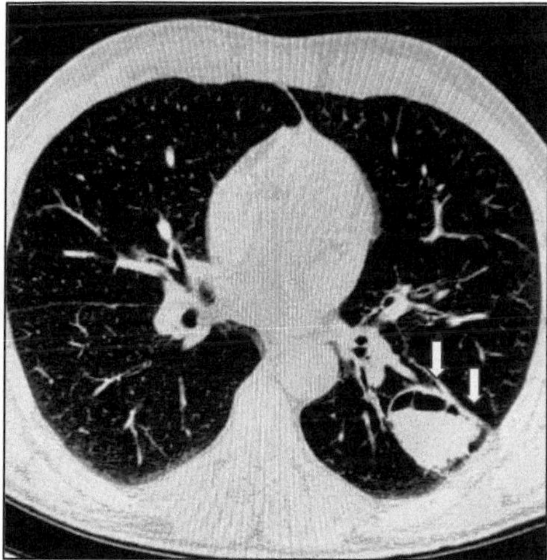

Figure9 Sagittal and axial sections of a thoracic CT angiogram in the parenchymal window in a patient presenting with massive haemoptysis showing a sequelae of tuberculosis in the apical segment of the left lower lobe with secondary aspergillus grafting.

1.4.2.4. Scannographic signs pointing to the bleeding artery

1.4.2.4.1. Frequency of different bronchial arterial anatomical arrangements

The growth of the bronchial systemic arteries was determined according to 4 types (Table XI).

Table XI Frequency of different types of bronchial artery births

Anatomical layout	Frequency N (%)
Right broncho-intercostal trunk (Figure10)	42 (72,4%)
Right-left common bronchial trunk	13 (22,4%)
Right bronchial trunk	1 (1,7%)
Left bronchial trunk	1 (1,7%)
Other variants	1 (1,7%)

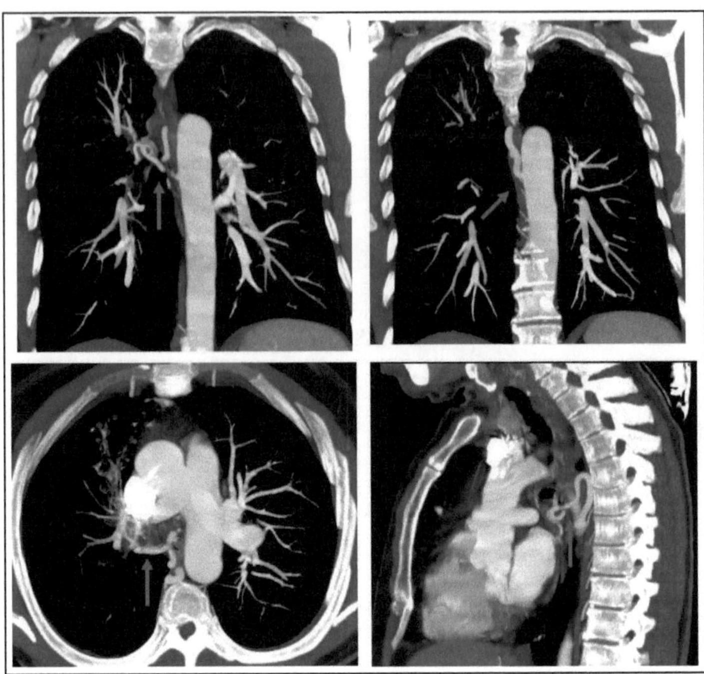

Figure10MIP reconstruction scans in 3 planes of space of a patient presenting with massive haemoptysis showing a dilated and tortuous right broncho-intercostal trunk (red arrows) responsible for the bleeding.

1.4.2.4.2. Bronchial arteries identified

After rereading the 58 thoracic CT scans, 84 identified systemic arteries were considered pathological. Fifty-five were bronchial systemic arteries (65.4%), including 40 orthotopic arteries (72.7%) and 15 ectopic arteries (Figure11), i.e. 27.2%. Twenty-nine (34.5%) were non-bronchial systemic arteries.

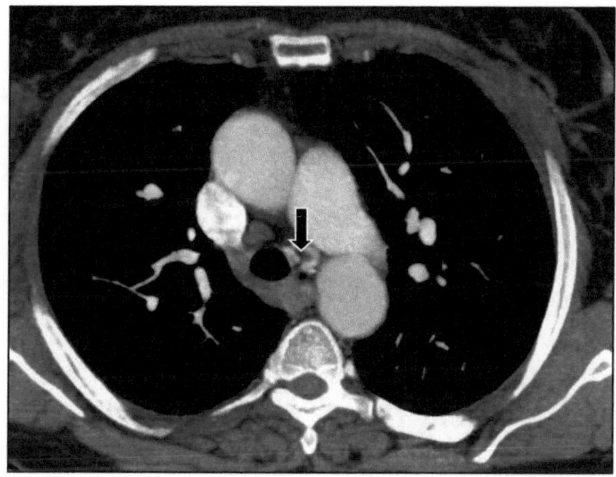

Figure11 Axial section in the mediastinal window of the CT angiography of a patient who consulted for massive haemoptysis showing an ectopic right bronchial artery arising from the descending aorta at D3. It was dilated and tortuous.

1.4.2.4.3. Characteristics of arteries considered pathological on CT angiography

1.4.2.4.3.1. Diameter

An ASB was considered dilated if its diameter was greater than or equal to 2mm. Straight ASBs had a mean diameter of 3.2mm with extremes ranging from 2 to 6.2mm. Left ASBs had a mean diameter of 3mm with extremes ranging from 2 to 4.6mm.

1.4.2.4.3.2. Ostium

The ostium of all the culprit arteries was identified on CT scan, i.e. 100% of cases (Figure12).

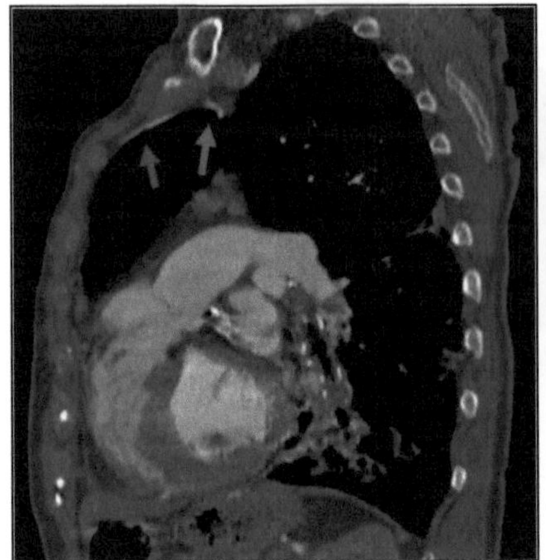

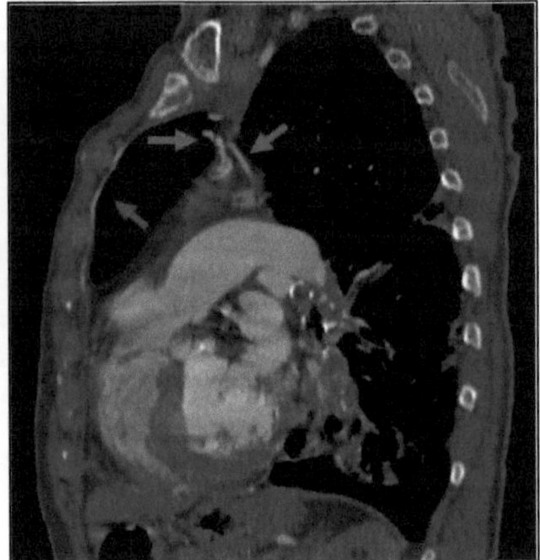

Figure12 Sagittal sections of a thoracic CT angiography in the mediastinal window with MIP reconstructions, of a patient who consulted for massive haemoptysis . It shows an ectopic left bronchial artery (red arrow) arising from the homolateral internal mammary artery (blue arrow). It is dilated and tortuous and joins the pulmonary parenchyma via the hilum.

1.4.2.4.3.3. Route

The course of the various pathological arteries was followed using CT. The results are summarised in Table XII.

Table XII: Traceability of pathological systemic arteries according to type

Arterial route	ASB - Frequency n (%)	ASNB - Frequency n (%)
No follow-up	0 (0%)	0 (0%)
Follow-up in the mediastinum	8 (14,5%)	1 (3,4%)
Follow-up in the hilum	24 (43,6%)	8 (27,6%)
Follow-up in the parenchyma	23 (41,8%)	20 (69,0%)

1.4.2.4.3.4. Tortuosity

The degree of tortuosity of the pathological arteries was assessed by CT. The results are summarised in Table XIII.

Table XIII Degree of tortuosity of pathological systemic arteries by degree of tortuosity

Degree of tortuosity	ASB - Frequency N (%)	ASNB - Frequency N (%)
No tortuosity	0(0%)	0 (0%)
Minime	12 (21,8%)	3 (10,3%)
Moderate	21(38,2%)	5 (17,2%)
Important	22 (40,0%)	21 (72,4%)

1.4.2.4.4. Retained artery responsible for bleeding on CT angiography

Our aim was to identify one or two of the most pathological arteries responsible for pulmonary hypervascularisation in each CT scan. These arteries were selected in 49 cases and considered to be candidates for EAB after review of the DTAs.

1.4.2.4.4.1. Type

We have divided these arteries considered culpable according to their type and side for each ATDM (Table XIV).

Table XIV: Distribution of culprit arteries for each CT angiography according to type and side .

Culprit artery	Frequency N (%)
1. Bronchial systemic arterial circulation	**38 (65,6%)**
a. ASB right	19 (32,8%)
b. ASB left	8 (13,8%)
c. Bilateral SBAs	11(19%)
2. Non-bronchial systemic arterial circulation	**6 (10,4%)**
a. **ASNB right** (Figure13)	3 (5,2%)
b. Left ASNB (Figure14)	3 (5,2%)
3. The two circulations	**5 (8,6 %)**
4. Not determined	**9 (15,5 %)**

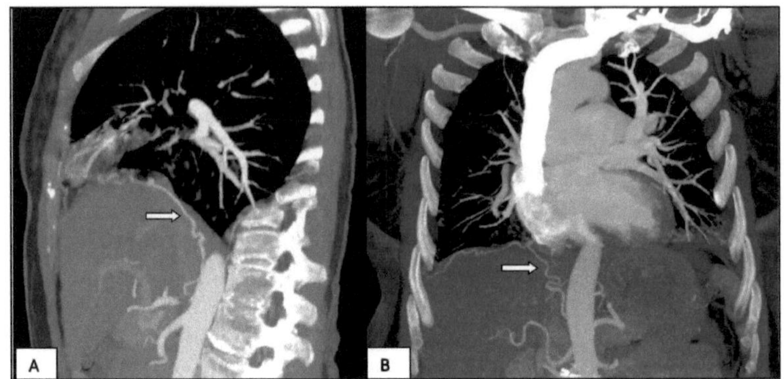

Figure13: Sagittal (A) and coronal (B) sections of a thoracic CT angiogram in the mediastinal window with MIP reconstructions showing a dilated and tortuous right inferior phrenic artery (Arrow) in a patient presenting with massive haemoptysis. This artery, considered culpable on CT angiography, was successfully embolised.

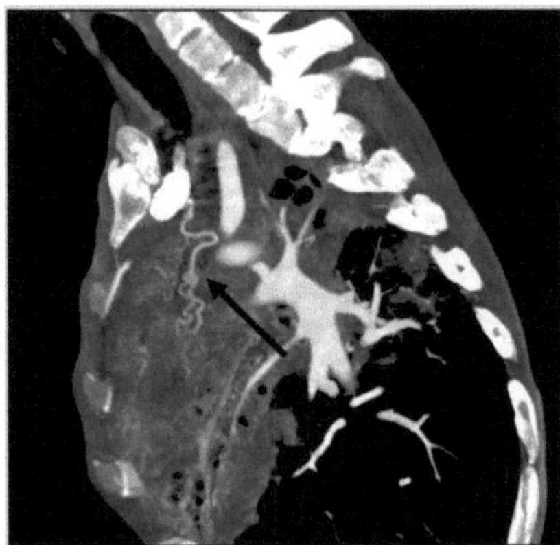

Figure14 Sagittal section of a thoracic CT angiogram in the mediastinal window with MIP reconstructions showing non-bronchial systemic hypervascularisation originating from the left internal mammary artery (arrow).

1.4.2.4.5. Detection of the anterior spinal artery on CT angiography

No ASAs were detected when the CT scans were re-read.

1.4.3. Bronchial angiography

All patients included in the study underwent percutaneous angiography for therapeutic purposes.

1.4.3.1. Angiographic signs

Forty-two patients (72.4%) had angiographic signs, which are summarised in Table XV.

Table XV Results of bronchial angiography .

Angiographic sign	Frequency (%)
Parenchymal blush	11 (19%)
Systemic pulmonary shunt	25 (43,1%)
Extravasation of contrast medium	3 (5,2%)
Pulmonary artery aneurysm	1 (1,6%)
Presence of an ASA	2 (3,4%)
No signs	16 (27,5%)

1.4.3.2. Artery considered to be responsible for bleeding on angiography

1.4.3.2.1. Visit

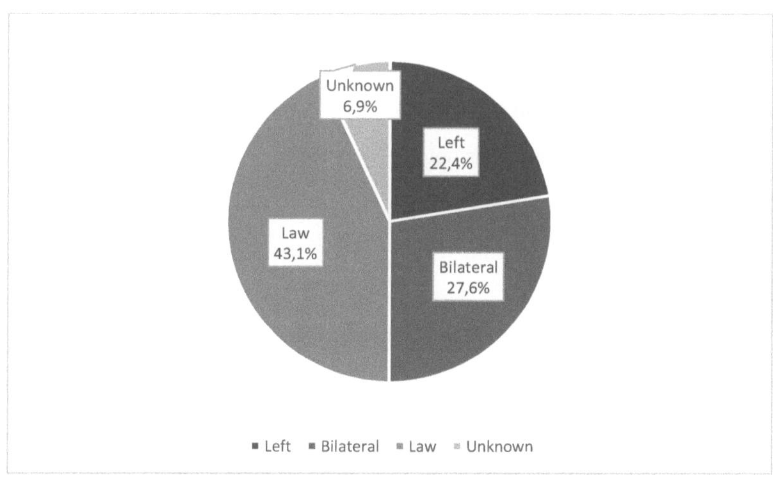

Figure15 Angiographic side of the culprit artery

1.4.3.2.2. Type

For each case, the culprit arteries detected at angiography were divided according to their type and side, as in DTA, in Table XVI. In cases where no culprit ASB or ASNB was detected, opacification of the pulmonary arterial circulation was performed.

Table XVI Distribution of culprit arteries for each angiography according to type and side

Culprit artery	Frequency n (%)
1. Bronchial systemic arterial circulation	**46 (79,3%)**
a. ASB right	22 (37,9%)
b. ASB left	8 (13,8%)
c. Bilateral SBAs	16 (27,6%)
2. Non-bronchial systemic arterial circulation	**5 (8,6%)**
a. ASNB right	2 (3,4%)
b. ASNB left	3 (5,2%)
3. The two circulations	**2 (3,4%)**
4. Not determined	**5 (8,6%)**

1.4.4. Bronchial artery embolisation

All patients were treated with EAB. In 55 cases, the bronchial arteries considered culpable on angiography were embolised. Embolisation of the right bronchial artery alone was the most frequent (n=17; 29.3%). In three cases, pulmonary artery embolisation was performed.

1.4.4.1. Embolizing particle

For each EAB, the particle used was noted (Figure16).

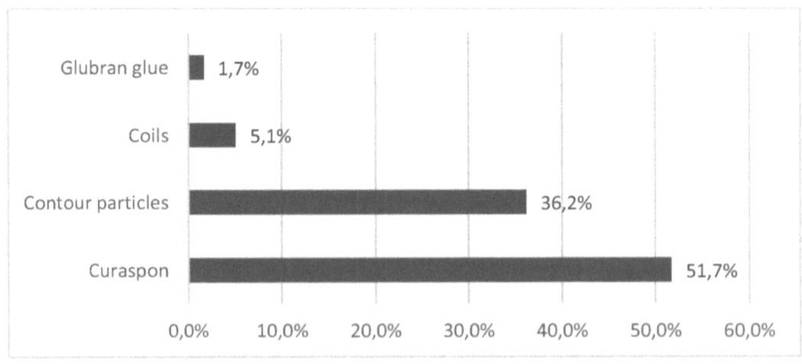

Figure16 Particles used in the EAB test

1.4.4.2. Results

1.4.4.2.1. Immediate success

Of the 58 embolisations performed, 54 were immediately successful (immediate cessation of bleeding), representing 93.1% of embolisation cases.

1.4.4.2.2. Recurrence

Recurrences were observed in 51.7% of cases (n=30): in the short term in 66.7% of cases (n=20), in the medium term in 30% of cases (n=9) and in the long term in 3.3% of cases (n=1) (Figure17).

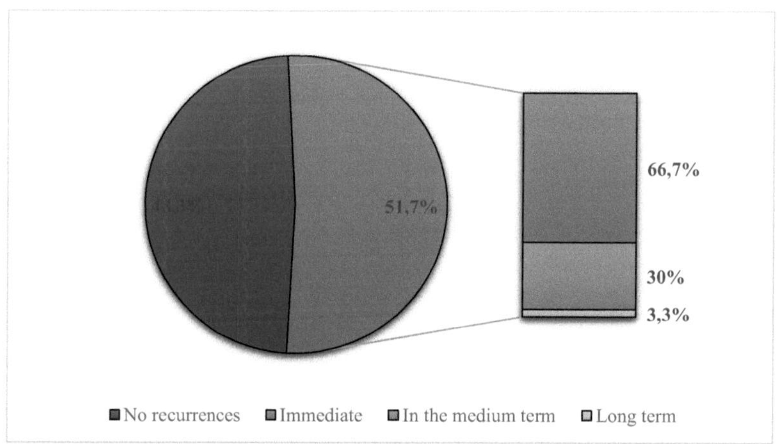

Figure17 Breakdown of patients in the group with recurrence of haemoptysis by time to onset .

The median time to recurrence was 2 months (IQR= [1-3 months]).

1.4.4.2.3. Complications

No major complications of EAB were noted in our patients. Only one case of per-procedural migration of coils (1.7% of cases) was noted, but with no subsequent significant consequences.

2. Analytical study

2.1. Role of thoracic CT angiography in determining the site of bleeding compared with conventional pre-embolisation angiography

2.1.1. Concordance of results between CT angiography and angiography

2.1.1.1. Stigmata of bleeding on CT scan and side of bleeding artery on angiography

We sought to find a relationship between the predominant site of bleeding stigmata on thoracic CT and the side of the artery judged to be responsible for the bleeding on conventional angiography. The results are summarised in Table XVII.

Table XVII Concordance between the site of bleeding on CT angiography and the side of the culprit artery on angiography

	Angio-Computed tomography	Angiography	Concordance	p
Bleeding on the right	26	25	17	0,999
Left bleed	17	13	8	0,424

No difference was found between the side on which bleeding stigmata predominated on CTAT and the side of the artery considered guilty on angiography.

2.1.1.2. Extent of bleeding on CT angiography and angiographic findings

No association was found between the extent of bleeding on thoracic CT and the presence of a systemic-pulmonary shunt or parenchymal blush on angiography (Table XVIII and Table XIX).

Table XVIII Extent of bleeding stigmata on CT angiography according to the presence of a shunt on angiography

	No shunt (n=25)	Shunt (n=21)	p
1-50% (1 to 10 segments)	17 (68%)	16 (76,2%)	0,539
51-100% (6 to 20 segments)	8 (32%)	5 (23,8%)	

Painting XIX Extent of bleeding stigmata on CT angiography according to the presence of blush on angiography

	No blush (n=38)	Blush (n=8)	p
1-50% (1 to 10 segments)	28 (73,7%)	5 (62,5%)	
51-100% (6 to 20 segments)	10 (26,3%)	3 (37,5%)	0,539

2.1.1.3. Systemic bronchial arteries (SBAs) responsible for bleeding

Concordance of the systemic bronchial artery culprit of bleeding between thoracic CT and angiography was observed in 42 cases (91.3%) out of a total of 46 cases (Table XX)(Figure18).

Table XX Concordance between CT angiography and angiography in the detection of ASB causing bleeding

		Angiography		Total	p
		Yes	No		
Angiomodensitometry	Yes	42	3	**45**	0,999
	No	8	5	**13**	
Total		**50**	**8**	**58**	

No difference was found between the two techniques in the detection of guilty ASB.

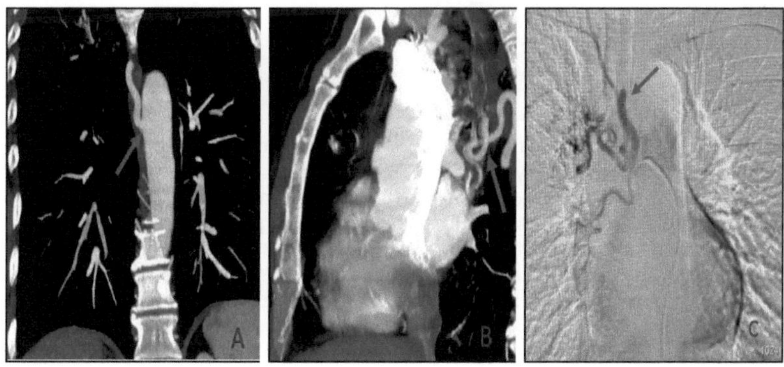

Figure18 Coronal (A) and sagittal (B) CT angiography sections with MIP reconstructions and an agiographic section (C) showing the ostium and path of a dilated and tortuous right ASB and an agiographic section (C) after selective catheterisation of this culprit artery confirming the CT findings.

2.1.1.4. Systemic bronchial arteries (ASNB) responsible for bleeding

Concordance of the non-bronchial systemic bronchial artery responsible for the bleeding between thoracic CT and angiography was observed in 4 cases (80%) out of a total of 5 cases (Table XXI) (Figure 19).

Table XXI Concordance between CT angiography and angiography in the detection of ASNB causing bleeding

		Angiography		Total	p
		Yes	No		
Angiomodensitometry	Yes	4	8	**12**	0,999
	No	1	45	**46**	
Total		**5**	**53**	**58**	

No difference was found between the two techniques in the detection of culpable ASNB.

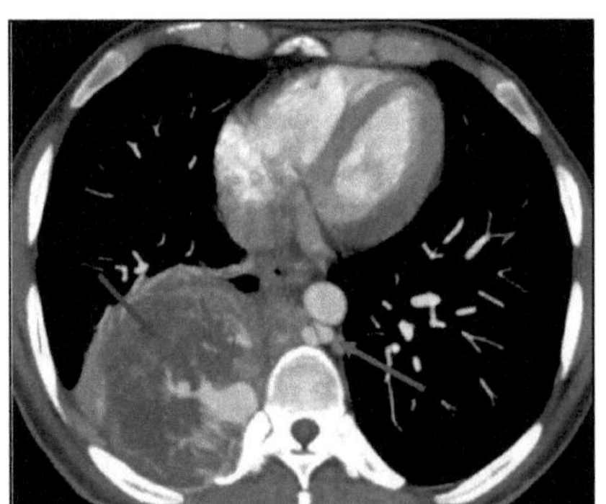
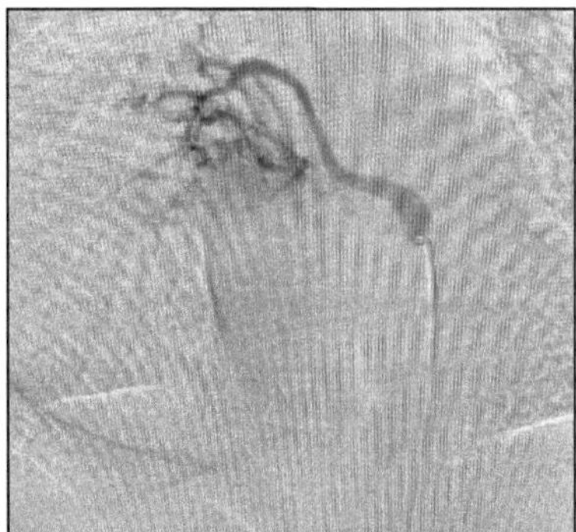

Figure 19 Axial section of a thoracic CT angiogram in the mediastinal window and angiographic section in a 37-year-old male patient consulted for massive haemoptysis showing a hypervascularised tissue mass in the right lower lobe (blue arrow). The hypervascularisation was systemic, not bronchial, originating from the 8 and 10 homolateral intercostal arteries, which were dilated and tortuous (red arrows). Selective catheterisation of these culprit arteries was performed successfully. Angiography showed pathological intercostal arteries.

2.1.1.5. Concurrent damage to both traffic systems

In two cases of simultaneous involvement of both circulatory systems on angiography, there was only one concordance with the results of DTA (p=0.375).

ATDM was superior to angiography in the detection of pathological ASNB associated with ASB in 4 cases.

2.1.2. Performance of CT angiography compared with pre-embolisation angiography in the assessment of pathological arteries

2.1.2.1. Systemic bronchial arteries (SBA)

TDCT had a sensitivity of 84% and a specificity of 62.5% in detecting the systemic bronchial arteries responsible for the bleeding compared with angiography.

Of these 42 cases of agreement between CTMA and angiography, the number of arteries was the same in 35 cases (83.3%), estimated to be greater than CTMA in 2 cases (4.8%) and less in 5 cases (11.9%).

There was no difference in the number of ASBs detected (p=0.527) (Table XXII).

Thoracic DTA performed as well as conventional angiography in detecting all pathological ASB (p=0.527).

2.1.2.2. Non-bronchial systemic arteries (ASNB)

Compared with angiography, DTA had a sensitivity of 80% and a specificity of 84.9% for detecting the non-bronchial systemic arteries responsible for the bleeding. Among the 4 cases of concordance between CTAT and angiography, the number of arteries was the same in 3 cases (75%) and estimated to be greater than CTAT in only one case (25%). There was no difference in the number of ASNBs detected (p=0.317) (Table XXII).

Thoracic DTA was as effective as angiography in detecting all pathological ASNBs.

Table XXII Performance of CT angiography in identifying the number of pathological arteries

	Angiomodensitometry	Angiography	P
ASB (n=42)	1 [1-1]	3 [1,25-4]	0,527
ASNB (n=4)	1 [1-2]	2 [1,25-3,5]	0,317

2.1.3. Performance of CT angiography compared with arterial angiography culprit

A better sensitivity of ATDM (100%) was observed when detecting the culprit ASNBs, in particular the diaphragmatic and internal mammary arteries (Table XXIII).

Table XXIII Performance of CT angiography in detecting the various culprit arteries

	Sensitivity (%)	Specificity (%)	PPV (%)	VPN (%)
Left bronchial artery	76	90,9	86,3	83,3
Right bronchial artery	75,7	92	92,6	74,1
Common core	83,3	92,3	55,5	97,9
Intercostal artery	66,6	89,1	25	98
Diaphragmatic artery	100	96,4	50	100
Mammary artery	100	96,5	33,3	100

2.1.4. Correlation between the characteristics of the culprit artery on CT angiography and the angiographic results

Arteries with minimal tortuosity were significantly more frequent in cases where there was no systemopulmonary shunt on angiography (38.5% vs 13%; p=0.044).

No association was found in our study between the path of the culprit artery on CTD and angiographic abnormalities (Figure20).

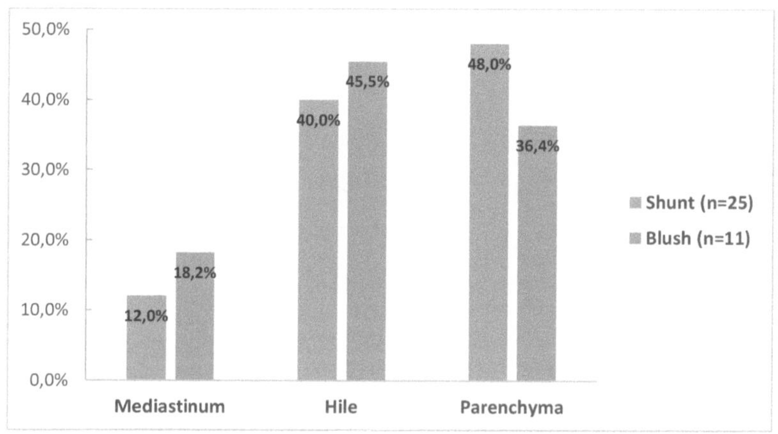

Figure20 Distribution of culprit arteries according to their characteristics and angiography results

2.2. Factors associated with recurrence of haemoptysis

2.2.1. Epidemiological factors

Recurrences were significantly more frequent in patients with a history of DDB (87.5% vs 46%; p=0.033) (Table XXIV). A history of DDB was a risk factor for recurrence (OR= 1.9; CI95%= [1.27-2.83]) (Table XXIV).

Table XXIV Epidemiological factors associated with recurrent bleeding

		No recurrences (n=28)	Recurrences (n=30)	p
Type	Male	22 (51,2%)	21 (48,8%)	0,456
	Female	6 (40%)	9 (60%)	
Age	< 60 years	17 (50%)	17 (50%)	0,754
	≥ 60 years	11 (45,8%)	13 (54,2%)	
Hypertension	No	19 (43,2%)	25 (56,8%)	0,169
	Yes	9 (64,3%)	5 (35,7%)	
Bronchial dilatation	No	27 (54%)	23 (46%)	0,033
	Yes	1 (12,5%)	7 (87,5%)	
Heart disease	No	25 (47,2%)	28 (52,8%)	0,467
	Yes	3 (60%)	2 (40%)	

Lung neoplasia	No	28 (50%)	28 (50%)	0,263
	Yes	0 (0%)	2 (100%)	
Pulmonary tuberculosis	No	26 (48,1%)	28 (51,9%)	0,667
	Yes	2 (50%)	2 (50%)	
Tobacco	No	10 (50%)	10 (50%)	0,849
	Yes	18 (47,4%)	20 (52,6%)	

2.2.2. Clinical factors

No relationship was found between the occurrence of recurrent haemoptysis and the time between diagnosis and treatment with EAB or between the occurrence of haemoptysis and EAB (Table XXV).

Table XXV Clinical factors associated with recurrence of bleeding

	No recurrences (n=28)	Recurrences (n=30)	p
Respiratory rate (Cycles/min)	15,82±1,517	15,9±1,729	0,855
Diagnosis/embolisation time (days)	4 [3-7]	5 [3-7]	0,844
Time between symptoms and embolisation (days)	7 [5-15]	7 [4-11]	0,775

2.2.3. Radiological factors

2.2.3.1. Chest X-ray

No radiographic sign pointing to the site or aetiology of bleeding was significantly associated with the occurrence of recurrence (Table XXVI).

Table XXVI Radiographic signs predictive of recurrence of bleeding

	No recurrences (n=28)	Recurrences (n=30)	p
Normal radiography	7 (38,9%)	11 (61,1%)	0,337
Pathological radiography	21 (52,5%)	19 (47,5%)	

• Signs pointing to the site of bleeding			
Alveolar syndrome	9 (50%)	9 (50%)	0,86
Interstitial syndrome	5 (83,3%)	1 (16,7%)	0,097
• **Signs pointing to the aetiology of the bleeding**			
Nodules	4 (100%)	0 (0%)	**0,048**
Micronodules	2 (50%)	2 (50%)	0,999
Atelectasis	0 (0%)	1 (100%)	0,999
Excavation	2 (50%)	2 (50%)	0,999
Round opacity	6 (66,7%)	3 (33,3%)	0,29
Spiculated opacity	2 (28,6%)	5 (71,4%)	0,425

2.2.3.2. Angio- thoracic computed tomography

2.2.3.2.1. Scannographic signs pointing to the site of bleeding

2.2.3.2.1.1. Scope

In the 46 patients who had signs of recent bleeding on CTAT, recurrence of haemoptysis was significantly more frequent in cases where the extent was greater than 50% (84.6% vs 36.4%; p=0.003) with an OR equal to 2.3 (CI95%= [1.4-3.8]) (Table XXVII).

Table XXVII Variation in recurrence according to the extent of bleeding stigmata on CT angiography

	No recurrences (n=23)	Recurrences (n=23)	p	OR	$IC_{95\%}$
1-50% (1 to 10 segments)	21 (63,6%)	12 (36,4%)	**0,003**	**2,3**	**1,4-3,8**
51-100% (6 to 20 segments)	2 (15,4%)	11 (84,6%)			

2.2.3.2.1.2. Predominantly

In our series, recurrences were significantly less frequent in cases where bleeding stigmata were predominant in a single left lung lobe (p=0.028). In addition, all cases of bilateral diffuse involvement or involvement of the whole right or left lung recurred after EAB (XXVIII).

Table XXVIII Variation in recurrences according to the predominant site of bleeding on CT angiography

	No recurrences (n=23)	Recurrences (n=23)	P	OR	$IC_{95\%}$
A right lobe	11 (55%)	9 (45%)	0,552	-	-
A left lobe	11 (73,3%)	4 (26,7%)	**0,028**	-	-
A right lobe and a left lobe	1 (50%)	1 (50%)	0,756	-	-
Left lung	0 (0%)	4 (100%)	0,054	**2,2**	**1,5-3,08**
Right lung	0 (0%)	2 (100%)	0,244	**2,1**	**1,5-2,8**
Diffuse	0 (0%)	3 (100%)	0,117	**2,1**	**1,5-2,9**

2.2.3.2.2. Scannographic signs pointing to the bleeding artery

2.2.3.2.2.1. Type of artery

Recurrences were significantly less frequent in cases where the right bronchial artery was responsible for the bleeding (p=0.037).

The risk of recurrence was significantly higher in cases where the ASNBs were involved (OR=1.6; CI95%= [1.04-2.5]) and in particular an intercostal artery (OR=2.2; CI95%= [1.6-3.1]) (Table XXIX). Recurrence of haemoptysis was significantly more frequent in cases where an intercostal artery was responsible for the bleeding (p=0.003) (Table XXIX).

Table XXIX Variation in recurrences according to pathological arteries on A CT scan

	No recurrences	Recurrences	p	OR	$IC_{95\%}$
Systemic artery bronchial tubes (ASB)	24 (53,3%)	21 (46,7%)	0,152	-	-
Systemic artery no bronchial tubes (ASNB)	3 (25%)	9 (75%)	0,07	**1,6**	**1,04-2,5**
Left bronchial artery	8 (36,4%)	14 (63,6%)	0,156	-	-
Right bronchial artery	17 (63%)	10 (37%)	**0,03**	-	-

			7		
Common core	3 (33,3%)	6 (66,7%)	0,272	-	-
Intercostal artery (Figure21)	0 (0%)	8 (100%)	**0,003**	**2,2**	**1,6-3,1**
Diaphragmatic artery	1 (25%)	3 (75%)	0,333	-	-
Internal mammary artery	1 (33,3%)	2 (66,7%)	0,526	-	-

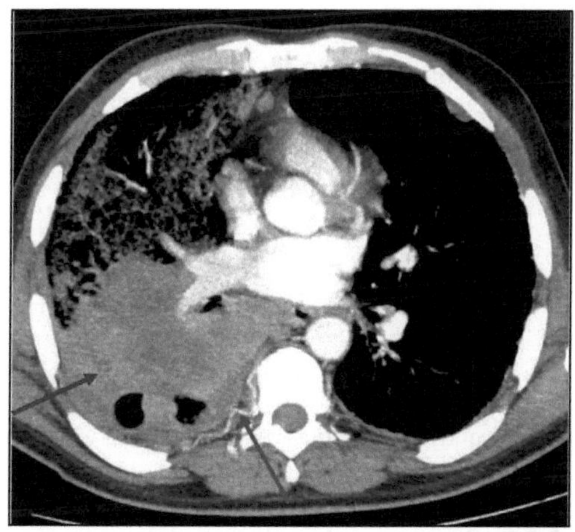

Figure21 Axial section of a thoracic CT angiogram in the mediastinal window with MIP reconstructions in a male patient who consulted for massive haemoptysis showing a suspicious lung mass in the right lower lobe (red arrow) and non-systemic bronchial hypervascularisation by a dilated and tortuous right intercostal artery (blue arrow).

2.2.3.2.2.2. Side of the culprit artery of the bleed

The frequency of recurrence of haemoptysis did not vary according to the side of the culprit artery when it was detected (49 cases) (Table XXX).

Table XXX Variation in recurrence depending on the side of the culprit artery

	No recurrences (n=23)	Recurrences (n=26)	p
Right	14 (50%)	14 (50%)	0,813
Left	6 (35,3%)	11 (64,7%)	0,203

Bilateral	3 (75%)	1 (25%)	0,344

2.2.3.2.2.3. Tortuosity of the culprit artery

Recurrences were significantly less frequent in cases where the arteries detected on CT scan had minimal tortuosity (23.1% vs. 61.1%; p=0.019) (Table XXXI).

Table XXXI Variation in recurrences according to the degree of tortuosity of the culprit arteries on CT angiography

Degree of tortuosity of culprit arteries	No recurrences (n=23)	Recurrences (n=26)	p
Minime	10 (76,9%)	3 (23,1%)	**0,019**
Moderate	8 (47,1%)	9 (52,9%)	0,845
Important	6 (31,6%)	13 (68,4%)	0,052

2.2.3.2.2.4. Traceability of the path of the culprit artery

Recurrences were significantly less frequent in cases where the path of the culprit artery was uniquely followed in the mediastinum (14.3% vs 57.1%; p=0.049).

2.2.3.2.3. Scannographic signs pointing to the etiology of the bleeding

The risk of recurrence was significantly higher if the pulmonary artery circulation was involved in the bleeding. In fact, all the cases of pulmonary embolism (OR=2; 95% CI= [1.5-2.5]) and the case of pulmonary artery aneurysm (OR=1.9; 95% CI= [1.5-2.5]) recurred after EAB (Table XXXII).

Table XXXII Variation in recurrences according to the frequency of associated signs

	No recurrences (n=28)	Recurrences (n=30)	p	OR	IC_{95} %
Nodules	3 (30%)	7 (70%)	0,178	-	-
Suspicious mass	4 (30,8%)	9 (69,2%)	0,152	-	-
Tuberculous signs	5 (71,4%)	2 (28,6%)	0,184	-	-
Tuberculosis sequelae	3 (37,5%)	5 (62,5%)	0,393	-	-
Pulmonary embolism	0 (0%)	2 (100%)	0,263	2	1,5-2,5
Parenchymal condensations	2 (66,7%)	1 (33,3%)	0,474	-	-
DDB	14 (46,7%)	16 (53,3%)	0,8	-	-
Parenchymal collapse	4 (50%)	4 (50%)	0,607	-	-
Rasmussen's aneurysm(Figure 22**)**	0 (0%)	1 (100%)	0,517	1,9	1,5-2,5

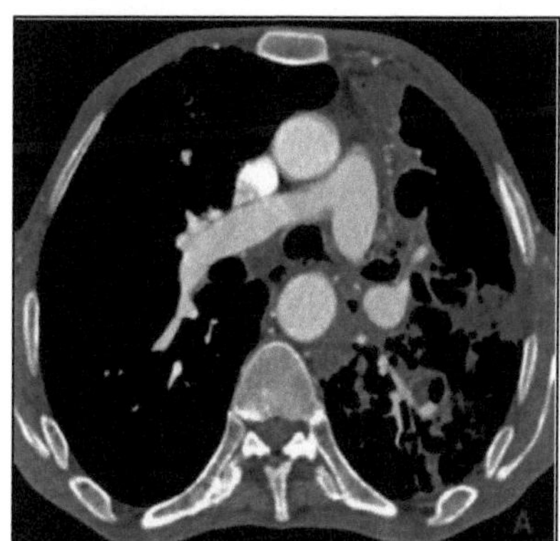

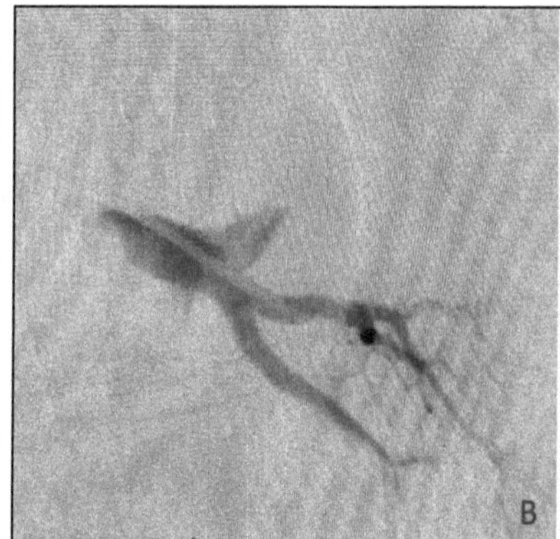

Figure 22 Axial section of a thoracic CT angiogram and an angiographic section of a 46-year-old male patient with active pulmonary tuberculosis complicated by massive haemoptysis.

A: Axial section in the mediastinal window of a thoracic CT angiogram showing a Rasmussen's aneurysm at the expense of a sub-segmental branch of the left Fowler's artery.

B: Angiographic section showing Rasmussen's aneurysm without extravasation of the PDC. This aneurysm was embolised with immediate cessation of bleeding.

No aetiology of haemoptysis was significantly more associated with recurrent bleeding (Table XXXIII).

The frequency of recurrence of bleeding was higher in cases of bronchopulmonary cancer and aspergilloma.

Table XXXIII Variation in recurrences according to etiology of bleeding

Selected etiologies of ATDM	No recurrences (n=28)	Recurrences (n=30)	P
DDB (Figure23 and Figure24)	12 (50%)	12 (50%)	0,999
Bronchopulmonary cancer	4 (30,8%)	9 (69,2%)	0,152
Active pulmonary tuberculosis	4 (66,7%)	2 (33,3%)	0,415
Idiopathic	5 (55,6%)	4 (44,4%)	0,726
Aspergilloma	0 (0%)	2 (100%)	0,492
Lung metastases	1 (50%)	1 (50%)	0,999
Pulmonary sequestration	1 (100%)	0 (0%)	0,483
Pneumoconiosis complicated by fibrosis	1 (100%)	0 (0%)	0,483
Pulmonary artery aneurysm	0 (0%)	1 (100%)	0,483

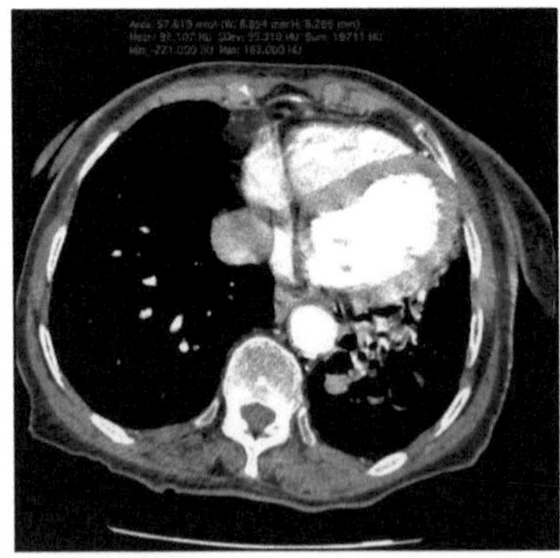

Figure23 Axial section in mediastinal window of a thoracic CT angiography in a patient presenting with massive haemoptysis showing left lower lobe DDB with endobronchial blood clots.

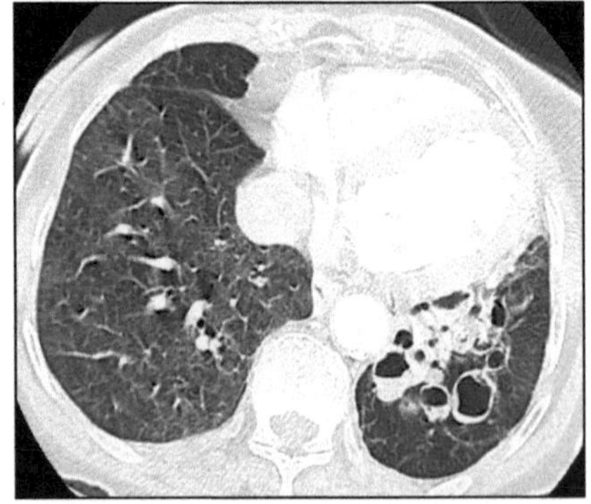

Figure24 Axial section of CT angiography of the same patient, in the parenchymal window. It shows partial filling of the pathological bronchi in the left lower lobe.

2.2.3.3. Conventional angiography

No difference in the frequency of recurrence was observed according to the presence of a systemic-pulmonary shunt (Table XXXIV).

Table XXXIV Variation in recurrences according to the presence of systemic-pulmonary shunt on angiography

	No recurrences (n=28)	Recurrences (n=30)	p
No shunt	17 (51,5%)	16 (48,5%)	**0,571**
Pulmonary shunt	11 (44%)	14 (56%)	

DISCUSSION

Over a period of 13 years and 5 months, from June 2008 to November 2021, we studied the records of patients admitted to the Pneumology Department of Mohamed Taher Maâmouri University Hospital in Nabeul and Sahloul Hospital for the management of massive haemoptysis.

All our patients were investigated by thoracic DTA in the medical imaging department of the same hospital and by percutaneous pulmonary angiography for therapeutic purposes prior to treatment with EAB in the diagnostic and interventional medical imaging department of Sahloul Hospital in Sousse.

Of the scannographic signs pointing to the site of the desired bleed, "ground glass" was the most frequent. In the majority of cases, the extent of bleeding stigmata was moderate or extensive and predominated in a right lobe of the lung. There was no significant difference between the site of predominance of bleeding stigmata on CT and the side of the culprit artery on angiography.

Among the parenchymal and mediastinal signs pointing to the aetiology of the bleeding, DDB was the most frequent. At the end of the diagnostic investigation, the etiologies of the bleeding retained, in order of frequency, were DDB, bronchopulmonary cancer and idiopathic haemoptysis.

We considered the bronchial arteries, which were tortuous and had an ostium identifiable on DTA and a tract that could be traced, to be the source of the bleeding. The results of DTA were consistent with those of conventional angiography in identifying the culprit arteries. There was no significant difference between the two techniques in the detection of culprit arteries.DTA had a high sensitivity and specificity in the detection of culprit ASB and ASNB. DTA was more sensitive than angiography in detecting culprit ASNBs.

After EAB, 51.7% of patients had a recurrence of bleeding, 66.7% of them in the short term. Recurrence was significantly higher when the culprit artery was a non-bronchial systemic artery, and particularly when it was an intercostal artery. The risk of recurrence was significantly higher when the pulmonary artery was involved. Recurrence was also more frequent when the stigmata of bleeding covered: more than 50% of the lung parenchyma, an entire lung field or was diffuse. Recurrence of bleeding was more frequent in cases of pulmonary aspergilloma and bronchopulmonary cancer.

1. Highlights of the study

- To our knowledge, this is the first national thesis to establish radiological criteria for recurrence of haemoptysis after percutaneous treatment with EAB.
- The DTAs were reviewed blindly and without knowledge of the angiographic data.

2. Weaknesses of the study

The methodological limitations of our work are :

- It was retrospective, with some clinical data missing and no radiological records, but this had no impact on the statistical analysis.
- The small number of patients was due to the fact that this is a rare condition and that treatment with EAB is only rarely available in Tunisia.
- The single-centre nature of the study.
- Prior knowledge of scan data before angiography.
- The final diagnosis made at the end of the various investigations was not histologically confirmed in all cases. However, the cases of bronchopulmonary cancer and aspergilloma all had anatomopathological evidence.

3. The role of thoracic CT angiography in determining the site of bleeding

Massive haemoptysis is a rare but serious condition that can be life-threatening with a high mortality rate. [12]. In this context, there are currently no clear recommendations regarding the performance of thoracic CT before percutaneous treatment with bronchial artery embolisation (BAA). The American College of Radiology (ACR), in its latest recommendations on haemoptysis, considers it to be "generally appropriate" for both massive and non-massive haemoptysis.[2,19]. Also, Cordovilla et al, in a study, suggested that it should be performed in patients with massive or recurrent haemoptysis[20,21]. In fact, several publications have suggested that thoracic DTA plays a crucial role in the positive and aetiological diagnosis of massive haemoptysis and consequently in preparation for treatment with EAB. They consider that it allows orientation towards the exact site of bleeding and the pathological artery. [12].

3.1. Scannographic signs pointing to the site of bleeding

3.1.1. Parenchymal signs of recent bleeding

In the past, the chest X-ray was the radiological examination to be carried out in the event of massive haemoptysis in order to detect signs of recent bleeding. It is still performed today as a first-line examination[22] given its availability and low cost.

However, it is normal or non-localising in 17 to 81% of cases of haemoptysis [23]. In our series, it was normal in 31% of cases and had a localising value in 41.4% of cases. It does not always lead to an aetiological diagnosis. In a series by Herth et al, 35 patients (24%) out of a total of 144 patients with bronchopulmonary cancer who presented with haemoptysis had a normal chest X-ray.[24].

In an article published by a Danish team in 2006, the authors suggested that a chest X-ray should be performed for a first episode of non-massive haemoptysis in the absence of two risk factors for lung cancer.[25]. If this X-ray is pathological, in the event of a recurrence of haemoptysis or in the presence of two or more cancer risk factors, investigation by thoracic CT scan and bronchoscopy is necessary.[25].

Bronchial endoscopy is still commonly performed in the event of massive haemoptysis. The use of a rigid bronchoscope is recommended in these cases. [8]. In our series, bronchoscopy was pathological in 78.4% of cases, oriented the bleeding side in 70.5% of cases and did not localise the bleeding in 29.4% of cases. In fact, in the literature, bronchoscopy is only useful in localising bleeding in less than 50% of cases[26,27] with a lesser aetiological diagnostic value than CTAT[8]. Chest radiography and bronchoscopy are therefore surpassed by CTAT.

Several publications have looked at the role of CTAT in the search for signs pointing to recent bleeding in the presence of massive haemoptysis.

It can show:

Initially, confluent centrilobular micronodules are seen, followed by areas of "vertrepoli" hyperdensity and sometimes parenchymal condensation. These abnormalities are predominantly central and inferior and spare the pulmonary cortex. [28,29].

In later stages, the interstitial sector is affected, with regular thickening of the septal lines and intra-lobular reticulations on CT. The combination of these signs with "ground-glass" hyperdensities gives a "crazypaving" appearance to the lung parenchyma. [28,29].

Areas of "ground-glass" hyperdensity and parenchymal condensation remain the most frequently encountered signs.[28,29]. In our study, the presence of just one of the signs described above was sufficient to localise a recent bleed.

We studied the frequency, extent and predominance of bleeding stigmata found. We then compared these findings with the side of the bleed on angiography. Signs pointing to the site of bleeding were present in 79.3% of our scans, i.e. 85.1% of pathological scans.

DAT was completely normal in 6.9% of cases, a lower percentage than that found in the literature, which is estimated at 13%. [30].

In our study, the extent of the signs varied from 1 to 19 segments, with an average of 6.6 segments affected. It was moderate in one third of cases, extensive in 24.1% and severe or critical in the remaining cases. In the vast majority of cases, it was localised to a right or left lobe of the lung, and rarely spread bilaterally or affecting an entire lung field.

In the literature, the most specific sign of localized bleeding is localized "ground-glass" hyperdensity images[1,11].

In the case of diffuse damage, the densest and least elevated area is considered to be responsible for the bleeding. [1]. The other scannographic signs related to the aetiology or consequences of the bleed were of lesser value in localising the bleed [1].

These data are consistent with those from our series, where there was no difference between the predominant location of bleeding stigmata detected on DTA and the location of bleeding on angiography.

In fact, in 70.7% of cases, the ATDM had a good value in localising the bleeding. Our rate is in line with the data in the literature (from 63 to 100%).[31].

In the same context, Seon et al studied 161 CT scans of patients presenting with massive haemoptysis. They found that the most decisive semiological elements for locating the site of bleeding on the CT scan were successively a specific lesion: tumour or fungus, an aspergilloma, or localised "ground glass" hyperdensities[12].

However, in the case of bilateral and diffuse "ground glass", it becomes difficult to determine the exact site of the bleeding. [12]. Indeed, certain aetiologies such as tuberculosis, bronchiectasis and pneumonia [12] result in bilateral lung parenchymal damage. This diffuse and bilateral involvement is generally indicative of a general systemic pathology and makes the patient a poor candidate for targeted treatment. [2].

In opposite cases, Seon et al concluded in their study of 161 CT scans that the predominant site of "vertrepoli" hyperdensities was the most specific sign for orientation towards the site of bleeding.

It should be noted that the consequences of bleeding, particularly endobronchial blood clots, can mimic or mask bronchopulmonary tumours, particularly endobronchial tumours or pulmonary nodules.[10]. Some authors require a scan to be performed at a distance from the acute episode [4].

3.1.2. Determining the etiology of bleeding

Determining the aetiology of haemoptysis is essential if the patient is to be properly managed. Surgery can remove the cause of the bleeding and is therefore the only radical curative treatment.[4]. However, it has a high mortality rate, estimated at 40%. [6,8]. In cases where the patient is not a good candidate for surgery, various medical and percutaneous alternatives are available depending on the cause of the bleeding [4]In addition, failure to treat the cause despite embolisation of the culprit artery in the acute phase exposes the patient to recurrence.[31]. Rebleeding in an already frail patient increases the risk of death from haemoptysis.

It is essential to distinguish between malignant and benign aetiologies, using CTAT. The mortality rate in cases of bronchopulmonary cancer or pulmonary metastases can reach 21% and is much higher than the haemoptysis mortality rate in cases of benign aetiology (5%). [31]. EAB is the treatment of choice for patients whose haemoptysis is due to a malignant cause [31].

In this context, ATDM plays a key role in determining the aetiology of bleeding, overtaking chest radiography and bronchial fibroscopy. [23]. It is particularly useful for diagnosing DDB, bronchopulmonary cancer and aspergilloma in cases of massive haemoptysis [23,31].

There are many causative pathologies for massive haemoptysis, and they differ from region to region. In developed countries, the most common causes are bronchopulmonary cancer, chronic inflammatory diseases of the lung, chronic obstructive pulmonary disease and aspergillosis.[4].

In developing countries, on the other hand, the most common causes of massive haemoptysis are active tuberculosis, sequelae of tuberculosis, in particular DDB, or aspergillary grafting on a tuberculous cavern. [4,23]. These lesions are generally diffuse and bilateral, and EAB is the most effective treatment. [4]. Rasmussen's aneurysm, which is a rare complication of pulmonary tuberculosis, can also be complicated by rupture, manifested by massive haemoptysis. [32].

Our results are consistent with the literature. The aetiologies of massive haemoptysis were DDB in 24 cases (41.3%), related to sequelae of tuberculosis in 8 cases (13.8%)

and associated with active pulmonary tuberculosis in one case (1.7%). A Rasmussen's aneurysm was the cause of bleeding in one patient treated for tuberculosis, and two patients had an aspergillary graft on a tuberculous cavern. Secondly, 13 patients had bronchopulmonary cancer (22.4%), one of which was associated with active tuberculosis. Two patients had pulmonary metastases. Nine patients (15.5%) had idiopathic haemoptysis with negative paraclinical tests. These patients underwent a second bronchial fibroscopy, at a distance from the acute episode, which came back normal. The remaining patients had rarer aetiologies, including one case of pneumoconiosis complicated by pulmonary fibrosis and four cases of acquired or congenital pulmonary and vascular malformations (pulmonary sequestration, abnormal venous return, bronchial arterial fistula, pulmonary arterial aneurysm).

In the same context, Chun et al studied a series of 50 patients hospitalised for the management of haemoptysis and treated with EAB at St George's Hospital in London. Their results were similar to ours in terms of the aetiology of bleeding, despite the fact that this study was carried out in a developed country. The most common cause of bleeding was DDB (16% of patients), followed by active tuberculosis (12%), aspergilloma (12%), bronchopulmonary cancer (10%) and pneumonia (8%). In eight patients (16% of cases), haemoptysis was considered idiopathic.[8].

Scannographic lesions pointing to the aetiology of haemoptysis can help determine the site of bleeding and the culprit artery. Given that any chronic pulmonary inflammatory process of infectious or tumour origin leads to vascular lesions by effraction or erosion causing bleeding. In addition, pulmonary bronchial arterial flow increases by about a third in the presence of a chronic inflammatory process [1,4].

3.1.3. Detection of the culprit artery

Several publications have shown that thoracic CT with its reconstructions in the three planes of space allows an exhaustive study of bronchial arterial vascularisation[31]. This facilitates selective catheterisation of pathological arteries and embolisation of the culprit artery during the therapeutic procedure[33,34].

3.1.3.1. Detection criteria

3.1.3.1.1. Diameter

Pathological arteries are dilated in the case of chronic inflammatory pulmonary pathology and have a diameter ranging from 2 to 3 mm [31]. However, they may be more dilated in certain pathologies, such as cystic pulmonary fibrosis [31].

In our study, we chose a cut-off of 2mm, above which an ASB is considered pathological. Right ASBs ranged in diameter from 2 to 6.2mm and left ASBs from 2 to 4.6mm, with mean diameters of 3.2mm and 3mm respectively.

In this context, Gupta et Al, who adopted the same cut-off in their study, found diameters on the right ranging from 2.2 to 4.3mm with a mean of 2.9mm and on the left from 2 to 5mm with a mean of 2.9mm.[34]In contrast, Yoon et al, using a cut-off of 1.2mm, found diameters ranging from 1.3 to 4.7mm with a mean of 2.8mm.[23]This is similar to the previous series and to our own.

3.1.3.1.2. Path and tortuosity

In our series, we studied the characteristics of all pathological arteries at DTA prior to EAB. We found that 40% of ASBs and 72.4% of ASNBs had significant tortuosity. In addition, 85.4% of pathological ASBs were followed at least as far as the pulmonary arteries and sometimes as far as the intra-parenchymal arteries. These data can be explained by the mechanisms and pathophysiology of haemoptysis. Indeed, any chronic inflammatory process leads to progressive destruction of the pulmonary parenchyma and systemic hypervascularisation[2]. As a result, pathological systemic arteries are dilated, tortuous and traceable on CT.

3.1.3.2. Type of culprit artery detected

Previous studies have also found thoracic CT to have high sensitivity and specificity in the detection of ASB and ASNB.

In one study, Pei-Jun Li et al searched for the artery responsible for bleeding on DTA by comparing their data with bronchial angiography performed prior to EAB[20]. The concordance between CT and angiographic data was 98.8%, i.e. 238 cases out of a total of 241 patients[20].

In our series, by comparing the scannographic data with that of angiography, according to the type of culprit artery :

3.1.3.2.1. ASB

Thoracic DTA had a sensitivity of 84% and a specificity of 62.5% for detecting pathological ASBs, with a concordance of 91.3% compared with angiography. This is consistent with the literature. Indeed, Remy et al found a CT/angiography concordance of 80% and Mori et al found a concordance of 86%. [33,35].

3.1.3.2.1.1. Ostium

Helical scans prior to EAB are performed over the entire thorax. It is used to search for the origin of the bronchial arteries: ASB and ASNB. In our series, we detected the ostium of all pathological arteries, i.e. 100% of cases.

Detection of the ASB ostium makes it possible to distinguish between orthotopic and ectopic arteries [12,33]. ASBs are considered orthotopic when their ostium is located at D5 and D6 on the aortic wall and ectopic outside this segment [13,14,23]. In our series, we detected the ostium of all ASBs. This is consistent with data from the study by Gupta et al who detected 100% of ostia in pathological bronchial arteries.

In our series, DTA detected 55 ASBs, of which 40 (72.2%) were orthotopic and 15 were ectopic (27.7%). Gupta et al detected 25 orthotopic arteries (92.6%) and 2 ectopic arteries (7.4%). [34]. In a series of 300 patients who underwent BAE for massive haemoptysis, Sancho et al detected only 25 ectopic arteries (8.3%). [15]. This is also consistent with the data of Yoon et al who detected 5 ectopic ASBs, or 9.6%. [23]This is in contrast to the series by Cohen et al, who studied 20 patients with cystic fibrosis complicated by massive haemoptysis and treated with EAB. They detected 7 ectopic arteries, i.e. 35% of patients.[36]. Remy et al found 4 ectopic right bronchial arteries out of 23, i.e. 17%, and 8 out of 30 left ASB, i.e. 27%. Li et al studied the clinical impact of performing thoracic CT before EAB in patients with haemoptysis and concluded that CT can detect more ectopic ASBs than angiography. [20].

In our series, the ectopic ASBs detected and considered culpable were easily catheterised and embolised.

3.1.3.2.2. ASNB

Several authors have described the need for a systematic search for ASNBs on pre-EAB DTA. In this context, several recurrences of bleeding after a first EAB were related to the persistence of bleeding through a non-embolised ASNB[20,34,37]In the series by Remy et al, three patients had a recurrence of bleeding after DES. Catheterisation of the ASNBs detected by the thoracic CT scan performed before the recurrence allowed treatment of the recurrent haemoptysis. CTA is useful for detecting pathological ASNBs feeding certain parenchymal lesions and thus responsible for bleeding. [12,34].

In other publications, the authors have reported scannographic signs that facilitate the detection of pathological ASNB. Pleural thickening greater than or equal to 3mm, especially in relation to parenchymal lesions, and enhancement of vessels in extrapleural fat [38].

In our series, we used these signs to review the CT scans. We detected 29 pathological ASNBs, i.e. 34.5% of all pathological arteries detected. In 11 patients (18.9%) of the 58 included in the study, six (10.4%) had normal ASBs and the bleeding was solely due to the ASNBs and in 5 cases (8.6%) both circulations were involved.In a series by Goh et al who studied the DTAs of 103 patients who had undergone BAE for life-threatening haemoptysis, 54 (52.4%) had pathological ASNBs. In 42 of these patients, both bronchial circulations were involved in the bleeding. The remaining cases had only the ASNBs responsible for the bleeding. Our data and those in the literature show that ASNBs are frequently implicated in bleeding during massive haemoptysis. They should be systematically detected on pre-EAB scans in order to reduce early recurrence of bleeding after EAB. [34].

In our study, CT had a sensitivity of 80% and a specificity of 84.9% in detecting the ASNBs responsible for the bleeding and was superior to angiography. Our data are consistent with those of the series by Yoon et al, where CT had a sensitivity of 80% and a specificity of 84%.

3.1.3.3. Pulmonary arterial circulation

Rarely, the origin of bleeding in massive haemoptysis is the pulmonary arterial circulation. In fact, in 90% of cases the origin of the bleeding is the bronchial arterial circulation, in 5% of cases the bleeding comes from the pulmonary circulation and in the remaining cases the bleeding may come from the aorta. [27].

Distal pulmonary artery bleeding is rarely serious [1].

The aetiologies of pulmonary arterial bleeding are pulmonary embolism, Rasmussen's aneurysm, arteriovenous malformation or direct arterial invasion by bronchopulmonary cancer. [34].

In our series, pulmonary arterial circulation was involved in haemoptysis in 5 cases (8.6%). In two cases we noted pulmonary embolism with pathological dilated bronchial arteries. In 3 cases (5.1%) the bleeding was solely of pulmonary arterial origin and the bronchial arteries were considered normal on angiography. One patient had a Rasmussen's aneurysm, which was embolised. One patient had a bronchial arterial fistula and the last patient had an abnormal venous return with secondary pulmonary hypertension.

In their series of 27 patients with massive haemoptysis, Gupta et al had only one patient (3.7%) with chronic pulmonary embolism involved in the bleeding.

In the literature, the presence of a pulmonary embolism represents a relative contraindication to EAB. In fact, it increases the risk of post-procedural ischaemic complications [34]. However, it remains unavoidable when the patient's vital prognosis is at stake [34].

In our series, the two patients with pulmonary embolism had massive haemoptysis and underwent emergency embolisation of the pathological bronchial arteries. We achieved immediate success in both cases, but the bleeding recurred in the medium term.

Opacification of the pulmonary circulation during EAB is not systematic. [39]. In our series, it was performed in the five cases where no pathological systemic artery was detected. The aim was to search for a pulmonary origin of the bleeding, which was found in 03 cases in our study. This is comparable to the data of Yu Tang Goh et al who performed only one pulmonary angiography in a patient who consulted for massive haemoptysis and who had agenesis of the right pulmonary artery, in a series of 134 patients. [39].

3.1.4. Other vascular anomalies

Certain rare congenital vascular anomalies, such as pulmonary sequestration, can be complicated by massive haemoptysis.[40,41]. In this particular case, thoracic CT can be used to detect and monitor the aberrant vessel and confirm the diagnosis [34,42]It confirms the absence of connection with the bronchial tree and pulmonary artery circulation and the absence of pulmonary parenchymal lesions. [34]. In our series, we detected only one case (1.7%) of intra-lobar pulmonary sequestration. The curative treatment for this condition is surgery. However, preoperative EAB can reduce the risk of intraoperative bleeding [2,40,41].

3.1.5. Detection of the anterior spinal artery

The presence of an anatomical variant of the anterior spinal artery (ASA) type communicating with the bronchial arteries may represent a contraindication to EAB. If present during embolisation, these collaterals may lead to spinal cord ischaemia and paraplegia[43,44]In our series, no ASA was detected on the pre-EAB scan. However, it was present in two patients (3.4%) and diagnosed on angiography. These two patients underwent hyperselective embolisation of the distal pathological arteries.

Our data are consistent with the literature. Admittedly, in the study by Gupta et al, only one patient had an anterior spinal artery that was not detected on CT and detected on conventional angiography[34]Furthermore, in the series by Remy-Jardin et al, no ASA was detected on DTA despite the MIP reconstructions performed. [33].

In our study, no major complications were noted after EAB, even in the case of per-procedural wire migration and the two cases of hyperselective EAB in the presence of an ASA. This is consistent with the data in the literature. In fact, the risk of post-EAB spinal cord ischaemia has now been significantly reduced thanks to super-selective catheterisation of the pathological arteries to be embolised. [31].

We conclude from these data that ATDM is not effective for the detection of ASA and cannot replace conventional angiography in this context.

3.1.6. Aortography

Some authors recommend that thoracic aortography should be performed systematically before any EAB in order to improve the detection of ASB and ASNB. [33]. Others have shown that, thanks to multi-planar reconstructions, CT angiography can provide high-resolution angiographic images [4,8,33]. In our series, no aortography was performed prior to EAB for the detection of ASB and ASNB. Catheterisation of pathological arteries was guided solely by DTA with three-dimensional reconstructions and MIP. Similarly, Yu Tang Goh et al did not perform aortography in 103 patients and opted for selective catheterisation of pathological arteries combined with angiography.[39].

In our series, immediate success of catheterisation was achieved in 54 cases (93.1% of EABs), and 64 ASBs and 7 ASNBs were successfully embolised. Similarly, in a study by Gupta et al, 4 arteries (16%) of the 25 pathological bronchial arteries were not detected by aortography but were detected and followed up by DTA.Thus, DTA can replace aortography in the detection of all the arteries responsible for bleeding in massive haemoptysis and the latter is not essential prior to EAB.

Finally, we conclude that bleeding stigmata, in particular localised "ground glass", are of good value in determining the site of bleeding. ATDM is effective in determining the aetiology of the bleeding, which makes it possible to pinpoint the location of the bleeding and to provide appropriate causal treatment to prevent recurrence despite a successful EAB. It can be used to assess abnormal bronchial vascularisation. It is a guide for interventional radiologists prior to EAB and helps in the selection of EAB equipment (catheter size and quantity of embolising material). [7]. It allows selective catheterisation of the culprit arteries without prior aortography. This shortens the procedure, reduces patient and operator radiation, increases the efficiency of the procedure and reduces complications. [7,20,34]It is also effective in detecting certain rare congenital vascular causes. We therefore recommend that it be performed prior to any EAB for massive haemoptysis.

4. Radiological severity criteria predictive of recurrence

After stabilisation of patients presenting with massive haemoptysis and determination of the site and cause of bleeding by CT scan. Percutaneous treatment with EAB was proposed for all our patients.

4.1. Bronchial artery embolisation

Practised since 1964[45]EAB is the most effective and safest treatment for massive haemoptysis, with an overall success rate varying between 82% and 90% in centres accustomed to performing this procedure. [7,46-48].

Admittedly, this is a palliative rather than a curative treatment because of the relatively high risk of recurrence of bleeding, which is higher than that observed after surgery.[6].

Recurrence of bleeding after EAB is due to incomplete embolisation, revascularisation of the embolised artery in 87% of cases according to Tanaka et al. [49]the development of collateral circulation or the evolution of the causal pathology, which has been ineffectively treated[46,50].

There are two peaks in the recurrence of bleeding after EAB: an early recurrence at one month, which accounts for 5 to 10% of recurrences; and an early recurrence at two months, which accounts for 5 to 10% of recurrences. [51]. This is due to incomplete EAB because the ASNBs have not been embolised. [52]. Long-term recurrence occurs after 1-2 years with a rate varying between 20 and 40% of cases in non-cancerous patients.[51]. It is due to hypervascularisation by progression of the causative pathology [52].

In our series, immediate control of bleeding was achieved in 93.1% of cases. This percentage is comparable to that of Springer et al [53]which was 95.75%, Chun et al [46]which was 86% and Ramakantan et al which was 73%. [3].

The recurrence rate was 51.7% in our study. This rate is comparable to that of Mal et al who studied 56 patients treated with EAB at the Beaujon Hospital in Paris and 55.3% of whom presented with a recurrence of bleeding during follow-up. [47]. Similarly, in a series by Fernando et al, the recurrence rate was 42.3%. [54].

Recurrence rates of haemoptysis after EAB vary in the literature from 7% to 55.3%. [46] and may reach higher rates in cystic pulmonary fibrosis [55]. This difference is mainly due to the length of follow-up of patients after EAB[47]the characteristics of the population (initial abundance of haemoptysis, patient's condition, clinical severity and aetiology of the bleed), the EAB technique and the embolising material used.

Most recurrences occur in the short term [46]. In our series, 66.7% of recurrences occurred in the first month of follow-up, 30% in the medium term (3 to 12 months) and 3.3% in the long term (beyond 1 year). These results are comparable to those of Chun et al who found 64.3% of recurrences at one month and 21.4% between 3 and 12 months.[46].

The high recurrence rate in our series compared to many previous studies [46] is thought to be due to the minimalist EAB technique adopted. In fact, for twenty-nine pathological ASNBs detected on DTA, only 7 ASNBs were embolised, i.e. 24% of the total. The early recurrences in our series are probably due to incomplete EAB as a result of failure to embolise pathological ASNBs. They correspond to the first peak described by Hayakawa et al. [52].

4.2. Risk factors for recurrence of bleeding

Previous publications have looked for risk factors for recurrence of haemoptysis after EAB. These predictive factors for recurrence were mainly related to inadequate aetiological treatment and the embolisation technique.

In our work, we tried to look for radiological signs predictive of recurrence even before the EAB was performed. Our main tool was the CT scan.

4.2.1. Identification of high-risk patients (epidemiology and clinical)

Before starting to treat patients with EAB, it is important to select patients at high risk of recurrence firstly on the basis of epidemiological data and then clinico-biological data. In our series, no relationship was observed between bleeding recurrence and patients' sex, age, cardiovascular history or smoking habits. This is consistent with the literature[6,46]. The only clinical risk factor significantly associated with recurrence was a history of previous DDB. To our knowledge, no other publication has found a similar result. In fact, we found in the literature other risk factors not studied in our series, such as, in the series by Kim et al, a personal history of chronic liver disease was a risk factor for recurrence.[56]. Also, Hwang et al found that type II diabetes was a risk factor for recurrent bleeding. [57].

Biological data were not studied in our series. However, some authors have found that a high level of C-reactive protein (CRP) in the blood can be a risk factor for recurrence. [56].

4.2.2. Radiological factors

4.2.2.1. Chest X-ray

No radiographic sign was statistically associated with recurrence of haemoptysis. Chest radiography has a role to play in the initial management of patients presenting with massive haemoptysis, as detailed above. However, it has no role in detecting factors predictive of recurrence.

4.2.2.2. A ngiotomodensitometry

Li et al have shown that performing DTA prior to EAB reduces the risk of post-procedural recurrence. [20]. This was also validated in a study by Zhang et al in 2020 [58]. In our work, all patients underwent DTA prior to EAB.

4.2.2.2.1. Extent and predominance of parenchymal bleeding stigmata

Several authors have found that the parenchymal extent of "ground-glass" hyperdensities correlates with the extent of bleeding and clinical severity [1,59]. We studied the occurrence of recurrence according to the characteristics of the parenchymal bleeding stigmata found. We found that recurrence was significantly more frequent when more than 50% of the lung parenchyma was involved, i.e. six or more lung segments (p=0.003). Similarly, we observed a significantly higher risk of recurrence in cases of diffuse involvement (OR=2.1; 95% CI= [1.5-1.9]) or of an entire right or left lung field (OR=2.1; 95% CI= [1.5-2.8] and OR=2.2; 95% CI= [1.5-3.08]). In fact, all the patients studied who had these signs on CTAT had a recurrence of bleeding. Also, recurrence was significantly less frequent when bleeding stigmata were limited to a single left lung lobe (p=0.028).

To our knowledge, there are no publications on this subject in the literature, and our data need to be verified by subsequent prospective studies.

4.2.2.2.2. Characteristics of the culprit artery

4.2.2.2.2.1. Type of artery

In our study, recurrence of bleeding after EAB was significantly less frequent when the right bronchial systemic artery was involved (p=0.037). Furthermore, the risk of recurrence of haemoptysis was significantly higher if an ASNB was involved (OR=1.6; CI95%= [1.04-2.5]), particularly an intercostal artery (OR=2.2; CI95%= [1.6-3.1]). In fact, all our patients with an intercostal artery responsible for the bleeding had a recurrence of haemoptysis. Our data are consistent with those of Yu Tan Goh et al, Lu et al and Li et al [39,60,61]These series all found that ASNB involvement was a risk factor for recurrence. To our knowledge, the only study that did not validate these results was carried out in South Korea on a series of 180 patients, all of whom had pulmonary tuberculosis and presented with haemoptysis treated with EAB. The difference may be due to patient selection bias.

4.2.2.2.2.2. Side of the culprit artery

We found no significant relationship between the side of the culprit artery and the occurrence of a recurrence. In fact, the risk of rebleeding remains invariable whatever the side of the artery responsible for the bleed. We did not find similar results in the literature. Our data therefore need to be confirmed by further studies.

4.2.2.2.2.3. Appearance and course of the culprit artery

We studied the calibre, tortuosity and traceability of the artery responsible for the bleeding. Recurrent bleeding after EAB was significantly less frequent when the arteries involved were not very pathological, i.e. when they had minimal tortuosity (p=0.019) and were traced only in the mediastinum. Furthermore, recurrence of bleeding was more frequent in cases of moderate (52.9%) and significant (68.4%) tortuosity. However, this relationship was not statistically significant in our study. In fact, we did not find a significantly higher risk of recurrence when the culprit arteries were very tortuous or were traced to the lung parenchyma. However, this relationship was demonstrated by Kim et al, who showed that recurrence of haemoptysis was significantly more frequent in cases of dilated and tortuous arteries. [56]. The difference could be explained, on the one hand, by the smaller size of our sample compared with that of Kim et al (58 patients compared with 190 patients) and, on the other hand, by the selection bias of their patients, who all had active and inactive pulmonary tuberculosis.

4.2.2.2.3. Scanographic signs pointing to the etiology of the bleeding

Several publications have shown that parenchymal sequelae of pulmonary tuberculosis are risk factors for recurrence of haemoptysis after EAB [56,61]. In fact, they constitute a chronic inflammatory process which maintains bleeding[61]. Although unproven in our study, we found that 62.5% of our patients with pulmonary tuberculosis sequelae on CTAT had a recurrence. This rate was not statistically significant in our series. This may be due to the small number of patients included in our series (eight patients) who had pulmonary tuberculosis sequelae on pre-EAB TST.

In our series, the risk of recurrence of haemoptysis was significantly higher if the pulmonary artery circulation was involved. In fact, all patients with pulmonary embolism (OR=2; 95% CI= [1.5-2.5]) or pulmonary artery aneurysm (OR=1.9; 95% CI= [1.5-2.5]) had a recurrence of bleeding. These results are comparable with data from previous publications [62].

4.2.2.2.4. Definitive etiology of haemoptysis

We assessed the risk of recurrence according to the aetiology of the bleeding selected after radiological and biological investigations. No aetiology was statistically significantly associated with recurrent bleeding.

However, in our series, the frequency of recurrence of haemoptysis after EAB was higher in patients with aspergilloma and bronchopulmonary cancer. Indeed, both patients with aspergilloma (100% of cases) and 69.2% of patients with bronchopulmonary cancer had recurrence of haemoptysis after treatment. These rates were not statistically significant given the small number of patients included.

Our data are consistent with those in the literature. Indeed,aspergilloma has a high risk of recurrence of haemoptysis ranging from 50 to 100% with a high mortality rate during the first month after an EAB [31]In fact, it is an aggressive process responsible for multiple pleural adhesions.[46]. Thus, the absence of surgical treatment or inadequate antibiotic treatment after EAB increases late recurrence between two and five years. [31]In the literature, the least favourable results of EAB were obtained with aspergilloma.[46]. As in our case, Chun et al in their series found 100% recurrence and 50% death in six patients with aspergilloma.[46]. In this study, the only statistically significant factor for recurrence was pulmonary aspergilloma [46]. These results were comparable to those of several studies [46,47,63,64].

For malignant aetiologies, Swanson et al and Hayakawa et al found that the highest rate of recurrence was observed in patients with malignant pulmonary aetiology [52,65]. Moreover, in the series by Hayakawa et al, the most unfavourable long-term results were observed in patients with pulmonary neoplasia [52].

As for pulmonary tuberculosis, the results found in the literature are discordant and differ widely from one team to another. In our series, active tuberculosis was not significantly associated with rebleeding. In fact, the lowest rate of recurrence in our series was found in patients with tuberculosis (33.3%). This rate was comparable to that of Ramakantan et al who found a relatively low immediate success rate (73%) in patients followed for tuberculosis and a recurrence rate of 27.1%. [3].

On the other hand, in a series of 103 patients by Yu-Tang Goh et al, the 16 patients who relapsed all had pulmonary tuberculosis and required a second EAB [39] In contrast, no non-tuberculous patients required a second EAB. Kim et al also found that the most common cause of recurrence was pulmonary tuberculosis [56]. Also, Lee et al found that bleeding recurrence related to chronic tuberculosis is greater than that due to DDB [60].

On the other hand, Kato et al found no recurrence of bleeding in patients with active tuberculosis. [66]. Also, Chun et al found the best results of EAB in patients with active tuberculosis [46].

In our series, the most common aetiology of haemoptysis was DDB. Fifteen patients (48%) with DDB had a recurrence after EAB. Our results are comparable to those of Hayakawa et al who reported 44.4% recurrences after EAB in patients with DDB. These results were the best in their series taking into account the aetiology.[52]. Similarly, Yan et al concluded that there was a lower risk of recurrence in patients with idiopathic DDB [51].

Nine of our patients had pulmonary haemoptysis that was considered idiopathic. Four of them (44.4%) had a recurrence of bleeding. In this context, Hayakawa et al had no recurrence of idiopathic haemoptysis after EAB [52]. This difference may be explained by the variation in the follow-up period, the variable abundance of haemoptysis and the characteristics of the population studied.

Other authors have considered pulmonary sarcoidosis as a risk factor for recurrence of bleeding after EAB. In fact, in a prospective American study of 69 patients treated with EAB for haemoptysis over a period of 11 years, Tom et al found that patients with sarcoidosis had a significantly higher risk of recurrence of bleeding.[67]. This factor was not studied in our series because none of the patients included had pulmonary sarcoidosis.

4.2.2.3. Conventional bronchial angiography

Conventional bronchial arterial angiography used to be the gold standard for the radiological diagnosis of massive haemoptysis. Since the advent of DTA and bronchial endoscopy, it has lost its place in the initial diagnostic approach. Moreover, it is considered "generally appropriate" in the ACR recommendations for massive haemoptysis and "may be appropriate" for non-massive haemoptysis. At present, it is only performed for therapeutic purposes and is the first step in any EAB procedure. [19].

It may show dilated and tortuous arteries responsible for bleeding[39]. The latter were more frequent in patients with recurrence in the series by Chun et al [46].

It may also show systemic-pulmonary shunts. In our series, no association was found between the presence of shunts and the occurrence of recurrence. This is consistent with the data of Kim et al [56]However, this association has been found in several other studies.[51,61]. In fact, the risk of repermeabilisation of a vessel after EAB was significantly higher in the presence of a sytemopulmonary shunt [61].

Angiography may rarely show extravasation of the PDCI. This anomaly was present in 3.6 to 10.8% of cases of massive haemoptysis. [31]. In our series, we found extravasation of the PDCI in 5.2% of cases. To our knowledge, no association between PDCI extravasation and recurrent bleeding has been found either in the literature or in our study.

Finally, clinico-radiological identification of patients at high risk of recurrence after BSE plays a preventive role. It allows selection of patients requiring closer monitoring and optimisation of management. [51]. In order to avoid recurrence in the acute phase, a complete BAE should be carried out, with embolisation of all the arteries considered culpable on DTA. Efforts should always be made to find pathological ASNBs. [39] as well as pulmonary arterial branches, and embolise them whenever necessary. Similarly, it is essential to treat the aetiology [46].

CONCLUSIONS

Massive haemoptysis is rare but serious, with a high mortality rate. It is defined as the release of blood from the lower airways when coughing. It is considered massive when the quantity of blood exceeds 300cc per 24 hours. It is life-threatening because of the risk of asphyxia. There is no consensus on its management. The aim of management of massive haemoptysis is to stop the bleeding in the acute phase and treat the aetiology to prevent recurrence.

Diagnosis is based on radiological examinations (chest X-ray and CT scan) and bronchoscopy. Chest X-rays are performed as a first-line procedure, but have a number of limitations: given their availability, chest CT scans are increasingly performed in the event of massive haemoptysis. It can be useful in determining the site of bleeding prior to percutaneous treatment and its aetiology in order to guide medical and/or surgical treatment.

The objectives of our work were to :

- To describe the role of thoracic CT in determining the site of bleeding in massive haemoptysis by comparing its data with that of conventional pre-embolisation angiography.
- Look for radiological severity criteria predictive of recurrence or mortality.

We conducted a cross-sectional descriptive study over a period of 13 years and 5 months, from June 2008 to November 2021, on 58 cases of patients presenting with massive haemoptysis and hospitalised in the Pneumology Department of Mohamed Taher-Maâmouri University Hospital in Nabeul or Sahloul Hospital, then investigated by thoracic CT scan in the Medical Imaging Department of the same hospitals and treated by EAB at Sahloul Hospital.

We included all patients with physician-confirmed massive haemoptysis who underwent thoracic CTD during hospitalisation and for whom percutaneous EAB was indicated. All these patients underwent pre-treatment bronchial angiography.

The mean age of the patients was 55.3 years, and the male/female sex ratio was 2.8. Sixty-five per cent of the patients were smokers, and 24.1% had a known history of chronic respiratory disease, mainly DDB (13.4%). Two patients had acute respiratory distress on admission. EAB was performed in all patients, with a mean time between onset of haemoptysis and EAB of 10.3 days and between positive diagnosis and EAB of 5.4 days.

The scans were read simultaneously by a junior radiologist and a senior radiologist.

We began by looking for scannographic signs pointing to the site of bleeding. CT scans were pathological in 93.1% of cases, with signs of recent bleeding in 79.3%. The average number of lung segments affected was 6.6. The extent was moderate in 32.8% of cases. It was located in the right lobe in 34.5% of cases and the left in 25.9%. DBDs were the parenchymal sign most frequently encountered, pointing to the aetiology of the bleeding (51.7%). The most common cause of bleeding was DDB, which was identified in 37.9% of cases. This was followed by malignant causes in 25.8% of cases and tuberculosis in 10.3%.

We then identified 84 pathological systemic arteries. The ostium of all these arteries was detectable on CT. All pathological arteries were traceable and tortuous to varying degrees on CT. For each patient, we considered one or two of the most pathological arteries to be guilty of bleeding and requiring embolisation. We then looked for concordance between the arteries considered culpable on CT and angiography.

All patients underwent pre-EAB angiography. A systemic-pulmonary shunt was present in 43.1% of patients. Nineteen per cent had parenchymal blush and 5.2% had extravasation of the PDCI.We found no difference between the site of bleeding defined on CT scan and the side of the culprit artery on angiography ($p>0.005$).Thus, CT signs pointing to the site of bleeding had good value in localising bleeding. The concordance between CT and angiography in the detection of culprit ASB was 91.3% and 80% for ASNB.there was no difference between the two techniques in the detection of the arteries responsible for the bleeding, whatever their type ($p>0.005$). ATDM had a sensitivity of 84% and a specificity of 62.5% for the detection of culprit ASBs and 80% and 84.6% for the detection of culprit ASNBs, respectively. ATDM was more sensitive than angiography in detecting pathological ASNBs, particularly the inferior phrenic and internal mammary arteries (Se=100%). We have thus confirmed, as in previous studies, that CTTA has a high sensitivity and specificity in detecting the ASBs and ASNBs responsible for bleeding. It can therefore guide the EAB procedure with selective catheterisation of the culprit arteries to be embolised without prior aortography. However, DTA was ineffective in detecting ASB in our study, and angiography should be used systematically to search for this contraindication to EAB.

Finally, we proposed to identify radiological factors predictive of recurrence of bleeding after EAB. Immediate control of bleeding after EAB was achieved in 93.1% of cases. We divided our patients into two groups according to whether or not haemoptysis occurred during the follow-up period. The frequency of recurrence of bleeding was 51.7%.

First, we identified patients at high risk of recurrence. Patients with a history of previous DDB had a significantly higher risk of recurrent bleeding (p=0.003).

Recurrences were significantly more frequent in the case of bleeding stigmata extending to more than 50% of the lung parenchyma (> 6 segments) (p=0.003). The risk of recurrence of bleeding was significantly greater in cases where an ASNB was involved in the bleeding (OR=1.6 and Ic25-95=1.04-2.5).

The risk of bleeding was significantly lower when the arteries were not very pathological, i.e. not very tortuous (p=0.019) and traceable only in the mediastinum (p=0.049). The frequency of recurrence was higher in cases of aspergilloma and bronchopulmonary cancer. Tuberculosis and DDB were not significantly associated with recurrent bleeding.

Finally, we have confirmed that DTA is effective in the management of massive haemoptysis. It plays a role in confirming the diagnosis and is essential in preparing for endovascular treatment and determining the aetiology with a view to appropriate curative treatment. We propose a standard report to be followed in the interpretation of the DTA in order to prepare the EAB procedure (Appendix 2). CTAT may enable us to select patients at high risk of recurrence of haemoptysis requiring close monitoring. We propose to confirm our results in larger, prospective, multicentre studies.

REFERENCES

1. Khalil A, Nedelcu C, Korzec J, Carette MF. Haemoptysis: pathophysiology and contribution of volume computed tomography angiography. EMC - Radiology and Medical Imaging: Cardiovascular - Thoracic - Cervical [Article 32-500-A-15].
2. Marquis KM, Raptis CA, Rajput MZ, Steinbrecher KL, Henry TS, Rossi SE, et al. CT for evaluation of hemoptysis. Radiographics. 2021 May;41(3):742-61.
3. Ramakantan R, Bandekar VG, Gandhi MS, Aulakh BG, Deshmukh HL. Massive hemoptysis due to pulmonary tuberculosis: control with bronchial artery embolization. Radiology. 1996 Sep;200(3):691-4.
4. Bruzzi JF, Rémy Jardin M, Delhaye D, Teisseire A, Khalil C, Rémy J. Multi-detector row CT of hemoptysis. Radiographics. 2006 Jan;26(1):3-22.
5. Ittrich H, Bockhorn M, Klose H, Simon M. The diagnosis and treatment of hemoptysis. Dtsch Arztebl Int. 2017 Jun;114(21):371-81.
6. Kim YG, Yoon HK, Ko GY, Lim CM, Kim WD, Koh Y. Long-term effect of bronchial artery embolization in korean patients with haemoptysis. Respirology. 2006 Nov;11(6):776-81.
7. Chen Y, Wang KF, Wang ZW, Liu CZ, Jin ZY. Value of CT-angiography in the emergency management of severe hemoptysis. Chin Med Sci J. 2019 Sep;34(3):194-8.
8. Chun JY, Morgan R, Belli AM. Radiological management of hemoptysis: a comprehensive review of diagnostic imaging and bronchial arterial embolization. Cardiovasc Intervent Radiol. 2010 Apr;33(2):240-50.
9. Cheah FK, Sheppard MN, Hansell DM. Computed tomography of diffuse pulmonary haemorrhage with pathological correlation. Clin Radiol. 1993 Aug;48(2):89-93.
10. Ramírez Mejía AR, Méndez Montero JV, Vásquez Caicedo ML, De Castro AG, Cabeza Martínez B, Ferreirós Domínguez J. Radiological evaluation and endovascular treatment of hemoptysis. Curr Probl Diagn Radiol. 2016 May;45(3):215-24.
11. Khalil A, Fartoukh M, Tassart M, Parrot A, Marsault C, Carette MF. Role of MDCT in identification of the bleeding site and the vessels causing hemoptysis. Am J Roentgenol. 2007 Feb;188(2):117-25.
12. Seon HJ, Kim YH, Kwon YS. Localization of bleeding sites in patients with

hemoptysis based on their chest computed tomography findings: a retrospective cohort study. BMC Pulm Med. 2016 Nov;16(1):160.

13. Cauldwell EW, Siekert RG. The bronchial arteries; an anatomic study of 150 human cadavers. Surg Gynecol Obstet. 1948 Apr;86(4):395-412.

14. Botenga AS. The role of bronchopulmonary anastomoses in chronic inflammatory processes of the lung. Selective arteriographic investigation. Am J Roentgenol Radium Ther Nucl Med. 1968 Dec;104(4):829-37.

15. Sancho C, Escalante E, Domínguez J, Vidal J, Lopez E, Valldeperas J, et al. Embolization of bronchial arteries of anomalous origin. Cardiovasc Intervent Radiol. 1998 Jul;21(4):300-4.

16. Clavier E, Douvrin F. Bronchial and extrabronchial embolisation in abundant haemoptysis. Reanimation. Mar 2006;15:61-7.

17. Marshall TJ, Jackson JE. Vascular intervention in the thorax: bronchial artery embolization for haemoptysis. Eur Radiol. 1997 Feb;7(8):1221-7.

18. Kettenbach J, Ittrich H, Gaubert JY, Gebauer B, Vos JA. CIRSE standards of practice on bronchial artery embolisation. Cardiovasc Intervent Radiol. 2022 Jun;45(6):721-32.

19. Olsen KM, Manouchehr Pour S, Donnelly EF, Henry TS, Berry MF, Boiselle PM, et al. ACR appropriateness criteria® Hemoptysis.J Am Coll Radiol. 2020 May;17(5S):148-59.

20. Li PJ, Yu H, Wang Y, Jiang FM, Wang W, Li XO, et al. Multidetector computed tomography angiography prior to bronchial artery embolization helps detect culprit ectopic bronchial arteries and non-bronchial systemic arteries originating from subclavian and internal mammary arteries and improve hemoptysis-free early survival rate in patients with hemoptysis. Eur Radiol. 2019 Apr;29(4):1950-8.

21. Cordovilla R, De Miguel BE, Nuñez Ares A, Cosano Povedano FJ, Herráez Ortega I, Jiménez Merchán R. Diagnosis and treatment of hemoptysis. Arch Bronconeumol. 2016 Jul;52(7):368-77.

22. Ong ZT, Chai HZ, How CH, Koh J, Low TB. A simplified approach to haemoptysis. Singapore Med J. 2016 Aug;57(8):415-8.

23. Yoon YC, Lee KS, Jeong YJ, Shin SW, Chung MJ, Kwon OJ. Hemoptysis: bronchial

and nonbronchial systemic arteries at 16-detector row CT. Radiology. 2005 Jan;234(1):292-8.

24. Herth F, Ernst A, Becker HD. Long-term outcome and lung cancer incidence in patients with haemoptysis of unknown origin. Chest. 2001 Nov;120(5):1592-4.

25. Andersen PE. Imaging and interventional radiological treatment of hemoptysis. Acta Radiol. 2006 Oct;47(8):780-92.

26. Hsiao EI, Kirsch CM, Kagawa FT, Wehner JH, Jensen WA, Baxter RB. Utility of fiberoptic bronchoscopy before bronchial artery embolization for massive hemoptysis. Am J Roentgenol. 2001 Oct;177(4):861-7.

27. Yoon W, Kim JK, Kim YH, Chung TW, Kang HK. Bronchial and nonbronchial systemic artery embolization for life-threatening hemoptysis: a comprehensive review. Radiographics. 2002 Nov;22(6):1395-409.

28. Jazzar MS. Hémorragie intra alvéolaire en milieu de réanimation: apport du scanner dans le diagnostic positif, étiologique et de gravité [thesis: medicine]. Tunis: University of TunisEl Manar; 2019.

29. Parrot A, Fartoukh M, Cadranel J. Alveolar hemorrhage. Rev Mal Respir. 2015 Apr;32(4):394-412.

30. RadchenkoC, Alraiyes AH, Shojaee S.A systematic approach to the management of massive hemoptysis. J Thorac Dis. 2017 Sep;9 Suppl 10:1069-86.

31. Ittrich H, Klose H, Adam G. Radiologic management of haemoptysis: diagnostic and interventional bronchial arterial embolisation.Rofo. 2015 Apr;187(4):248-59.

32. Mahmoud N, Moussa C, Attia M, Rouis H, Khattab A, Khouaja I, et al. Rasmussen aneurysm: a forgotten complication of tuberculosis in the COVID-19 era. Respir Med Case Rep. 2022 Oct;39:101714.

33. Remy Jardin M, Bouaziz N, Dumont P, Brillet PY, Bruzzi J, Remy J. Bronchial and nonbronchial systemic arteries at multi-detector row CT angiography: comparison with conventional angiography. Radiology. 2004 Dec;233(3):741-9.

34. Gupta M, Srivastava DN, Seith A, Sharma S, Thulkar S, Gupta R. Clinical impact of multidetector row computed tomography before bronchial artery embolization in patients with hemoptysis: a prospective study. Can Assoc Radiol J. 2013 Feb;64(1):61-73.

35. Mori H, Ohno Y, Tsuge Y, Kawasaki M, Ito F, Endo J, et al. Use of multidetector

row CT to evaluate the need for bronchial arterial embolization in hemoptysis patients. Respiration. 2010 Mar;80(1):24-31.

36. Cohen AM, Doershuk CF, Stern RC. Bronchial artery embolization to control hemoptysis in cystic fibrosis. Radiology. 1990 May;175(2):401-5.

37. Zhao T, Wang S, Zheng L, Jia Z, Yang Y, Wang W, et al. The value of 320-row multidetector CT bronchial arteriography in recurrent hemoptysis after failed transcatheter arterial embolization. J Vasc Interv Radiol. 2017 Apr;28(4):533-41.

38. Yoon W, Kim YH, Kim JK, Kim YC, Park JG, Kang HK. Massive hemoptysis: prediction of nonbronchial systemic arterial supply with chest CT. Radiology. 2003 Apr;227(1):232-8.

39. Yu Tang GP, Lin M, Teo N, En Shen WD. Embolization for hemoptysis: a six-year review. Cardiovasc Intervent Radiol. 2002 Jan;25(1):17-25.

40. Hoan L, Cuong NN, Thang ND, Hong DT, Hang LM, Linh LT, et al. A 24-year-old man with recurrent hemoptysis. Chest. 2020 Feb;157(2):31-5.

41. Kim TE, Kwon JH, Kim JS. Transcatheter embolization for massive hemoptysis from an intralobar pulmonary sequestration: a case report. Clin Imaging. 2014 May;38(3):326-9.

42. Do KH, Goo JM, Im JG, Kim KW, Chung JW, Park JH. Systemic arterial supply to the lungs in adults: spiral CT findings. Radiographics. 2001 Mar;21(2):387-402.

43. Di Chiro G. Unintentional spinal cord arteriography: a warning. Radiology. 1974 Jul;112(1):231-3.

44. Kardjiev V, Symeonov A, Chankov I. Etiology, pathogenesis, and prevention of spinal cord lesions in selective angiography of the bronchial and intercostal arteries. Radiology. 1974 Jul;112(1):81-3.

45. Viamonte M. Selective bronchial arteriography in man. Radiology. 1964 Nov;83:830-9.

46. Chun JY, Belli AM. Immediate and long-term outcomes of bronchial and non-bronchial systemic artery embolisation for the management of haemoptysis. Eur Radiol. 2010 Mar;20(3):558-65.

47. Mal H, Rullon I, Mellot F, Brugière O, Sleiman C, Menu Y, et al. Immediate and long-term results of bronchial artery embolization for life-threatening hemoptysis. Chest. 1999 Apr;115(4):996-1001.

48. Terlizzi V, Botti M, Gabbani G, Fanelli F, De Martino M, Taccetti G. Unilateral temporary diaphragmatic paralysis secondary to bronchial artery embolization in a girl with cystic fibrosis and massive hemoptysis: a case report. BMC Pulm Med. 2020 Feb;20(1):38.

49. Tanaka N, Yamakado K, Murashima S, Takeda K, Matsumura K, Nakagawa T, et al. Superselective bronchial artery embolization for hemoptysis with a coaxial microcatheter system. J Vasc Interv Radiol. 1997 Jan;8(1):65-70.

50. Bhalla A, Kandasamy D, Veedu P, Veedu A, Gamanagatti S. A retrospective analysis of 334 cases of hemoptysis treated by bronchial artery embolization. Oman Med J. 2015 Mar;30(2):119-28.

51. Yan HT, Lu GD, Huang XZ, Zhang DZ, Ge KY, Zhang JX, et al. Development of a model to predict recurrence after bronchial artery embolization for non-cancer related hemoptysis. BMC Pulm Med. 2021 Dec;21(1):419.

52. Hayakawa K, Tanaka F, Torizuka T, Mitsumori M, Okuno Y, Matsui A, et al. Bronchial artery embolization for hemoptysis: immediate and long-term results. Cardiovasc Intervent Radiol. 1992 May;15(3):154-8.

53. Springer DM, Cofta S, Juszkat R, Żabicki B, Goździk Spychalska J, Nowicka A, et al. The effectiveness of bronchial artery embolisation in patients with haemoptysis. Adv Respir Med. 2018 Jan;86(5):220-6.

54. Fernando HC, Stein M, Benfield JR, Link DP. Role of bronchial artery embolization in the management of hemoptysis. Arch Surg. 1998 Aug;133(8):862-6.

55. Flight WG, Barry PJ, Bright Thomas RJ, Butterfield S, Ashleigh R, Jones AM. Outcomes following bronchial artery embolisation for haemoptysis in cystic fibrosis. Cardiovasc Intervent Radiol. 2017 Aug;40(8):1164-8.

56. Kim SW, Lee SJ, Ryu YJ, Lee JH, Chang JH, Shim SS, et al. Prognosis and predictors of rebleeding after bronchial artery embolization in patients with active or inactive pulmonary tuberculosis. Lung. 2015 Aug;193(4):575-81.

57. Hwang HG, Lee HS, Choi JS, Seo KH, Kim YH, Na JO. Risk factors influencing rebleeding after bronchial artery embolization on the management of hemoptysis associated with pulmonary tuberculosis. Tuberc Respir Dis. 2013 Mar;74(3):111-9.

58. Zhang J, Zheng L, Zhao T, Huang S, Hu W. A retrospective analysis of risk factors in recurrent hemoptysis patients with non-bronchial systematic artery feeding.Ann Transl Med. 2020 Dec;8(23):1593.

59. Khalil A, Soussan M, Mangiapan G, Fartoukh M, Parrot A, Carette MF. Utility of high-resolution chest CT scan in the emergency management of haemoptysis in the intensive care unit: severity, localization and aetiology. Br J Radiol. 2007 Jan;80(949):21-5.

60. Lee JH, Kwon SY, Yoon HI, Yoon CJ, Lee KW, Kang SG, et al. Haemoptysis due to chronic tuberculosis vs. bronchiectasis: comparison of long-term outcome of arterial embolisation. Int J Tuberc Lung Dis. 2007 Jul;11(7):781-7.

61. Lu GD, Zu QQ, Zhang JX, Zhou CG, Xia JG, Ye W, et al. Risk factors contributing to early and late recurrence of haemoptysis after bronchial artery embolisation. Int J Tuberc Lung Dis. 2018 Feb;22(2):230-5.

62. Shin S, Shin TB, Choi H, Choi JS, Kim YH, Kim CW, et al. Peripheral pulmonary arterial pseudoaneurysms: therapeutic implications of endovascular treatment and angiographic classifications. Radiology. 2010 Aug;256(2):656-64.

63. Racil H, Rajhi H, Ben Naceur R, Chabbou A, Bouecha H, Mnif N. Endovascular treatment of haemoptysis: medium and long-term assessment. Diagn Interv Imaging. 2013 Jan;94(1):38-44.

64. Le HY, Le VN, Pham NH, Phung AT, Nguyen TT, Do Q. Value of multidetector computed tomography angiography before bronchial artery embolization in hemoptysis management and early recurrence prediction: a prospective study. BMC Pulm Med. 2020 Aug;20(1):231.

65. Swanson KL, Johnson CM, Prakash US, McKusick MA, Andrews JC, Stanson AW. Bronchial artery embolization: experience with 54 patients. Chest. 2002 Mar;121(3):789-95.

66. Kato A, Kudo S, Matsumoto K, Fukahori T, Shimizu T, Uchino A, et al. Bronchial artery embolization for hemoptysis due to benign diseases: immediate and long-term results. Cardiovasc Intervent Radiol. 2000 Sep;23(5):351-7.

67. Tom LM, Palevsky HI, Holsclaw DS, Trerotola SO, Dagli M, Mondschein JI, et al. Recurrent bleeding, survival, and longitudinal pulmonary function following bronchial artery embolization for hemoptysis in a U.S. adult population. J Vasc Interv Radiol. 2015 Dec;26(12):1806-13.

APPENDIX

Appendix 1

Analytical sheet

Patient data :

1. File number :
2. Full name :
3. Sex: M= □ ; F= □
4. Age :
5. Level of schooling: no schooling = □; Primary = □; Secondary = □; Higher = □.
6. Socio-economic conditions: Poor = □; Average = □; Good = □.

Personal history :

7. HTA= □ ; Cardiopathy= □ ; DDB= □ ; Tuberculosis= □ ; Neoplasia= □

Habits :

8. Smoking: Yes = □; No = □

Clinical data :

9. Date of hospitalisation :
10. Initial respiratory distress: Yes = □; No = □
11. Hemorrhagic shock: Yes = □; No = □
12. Oxygen saturation :
13. Time between diagnosis and EAB :
14. Time between haemoptysis and EAB :

Data from bronchial endoscopy :

15. Normal = □ ; pathological = □ ; not done = □.
16. Bleeding: No = □; Yes = □.
17. Bleeding site: unknown = □; AB right = □; AB left= □.
18. Stopped gesture: No = □; Yes = □.
19. Full exploration: No = □; Yes = □.
20. Fibroscopy redone at a distance: No = □; Yes = □.

Imaging data :

Chest X-ray :

21. Normal = □ ; pathological = □
22. Alveolar syndrome: No = □; Unilateral = □; Bilateral = □.
23. Interstitial syndrome: No = □; Yes = □.
24. Nodules: No = □; Yes = □.
25. Micronodules: No = □; Yes = □.
26. Atelectasis: No = □; Yes = □.
27. Excavation: No = □; Yes = □.
28. Round opacity: No = □ ; proximal = □ ; distal = □.
29. Spiculated opacity: No = □; proximal = □; distal = □.

Chest CT scan data :

30. ATDM appearance: normal = □ ; pathological = □

- Signs pointing to the site of bleeding:

31. No = □; Yes = □.
32. Extent: Absent = □
    1-25% or 1 to 5 segments = □.
    26-50% or 6 to 10 segments = □.
    51-75% or 6 to 15 segments = □.
    76-100% or 16 to 20 segments = □.
33. Predominance:1 = One right lobe = □.
    2 = One left lobe = □.
    3 = One right lobe and one left lobe = □.
    4 = Right lung = □.
    5 = Left lung = □.
    6 = Diffuse = □.

- Signs pointing to the etiology of the bleeding :

34. Presence of nodule: No = □ ; Yes = □.
35. Suspicious mass: No = □; Yes = □.
36. Active tuberculosis: No = □; Yes = □.
37. Sequelae of tuberculosis: No = □; Yes = □.
38. Presence of pulmonary embolism: No = □; Yes = □.
39. Presence of pulmonary fibrosis: No = □; Yes = □.
40. Presence of non-systematic condensation: No = □; Yes = □.
41. DDB : No = □ ; Yes = □.
42. Presence of pulmonary collapse: No = □ ; Yes = □.
43. The etiology chosen for ATDM :

- Signs pointing to the bleeding artery :

44. Number of pathological ASB (systemic bronchial artery) identified.
    a. Number of orthotopic arteries identified.
    b. Number of ectopic arteries identified.
45. Number of pathological ASNBs (non-bronchial systemic arteries) identified.
46. Birth of the bronchial arteries.
    1 = TBIC Right = □.
    2 = Common bronchial trunk = □.
    3 = Right bronchial trunk = □.
    4 = Left bronchial trunk = □.
    5 = other variants= □.
47. Ostium: Not seen = □; Seen = □.
48. Diameter of the culprit artery if known.
49. Path of the culprit artery: 0 = Not followed = □.
    1 = follow-up in the mediastinum = □.
    2 = followed in the hilum = □.
    3 = follow-up in the parenchyma = □.
50. Degree of tortuosity: 0 = no tortuosity = □
    1 = minimal = □.

2 = moderate = □.
3 = important = □.

51. Artery considered responsible for bleeding :
52. Presence of an anterior spinal artery: No = □; Yes = □.

Data from bronchial angiography :

53. Number of ASB bleeding
54. Number of ASNBs bleeding
55. Artery considered responsible for bleeding
56. Side and type of artery responsible for bleeding
57. Parenchymal blush: No = □; Yes = □.
58. Systemic pulmonary shunt: No = □; Yes = □.
59. Extravasation of CIDP: No = □; Yes = □.

Bronchial artery embolisation :

60. Embolisation : Not done = □ ; done = □.
61. Type of catheter :
62. Embolised artery :
63. Embolisation particle: 1 = curaspon(haemostatic sponge) = □.
2 = spongel = □.
3 = contour particles = □.
4 = polyvinyl alcohol particles = □.
5 = coils = □.

Evolution :

64. Immediate success: No = □; Yes = □.
65. Failure: No = □; Yes = □.
66. Recurrence: No = □; immediate = □, medium term = □, long term = □.
67. Time limit for repeat offences :
68. Overall survival.
69. Date of last consultation.
70. Total length of hospital stay.
71. Length of hospitalisation before embolisation.
72. Length of hospitalisation after embolisation.

Appendix 2

STANDARD REPORT: THORACIC ANGIOSCANNER

INDICATION :

Massive haemoptysis. Pre-embolisation bronchial artery assessment.

TECHNICAL :

RESULTS :

1- Pleuro-parenchymal and parietal study :

- Signs pointing to the site of bleeding: "frosted glass", parenchymal condensations or "crazy paving" appearance.
    - Extent: moderate, extensive, severe or critical, specifying the number of segments affected.
    - Predominant location.

- Signs pointing to the aetiology of the bleeding: nodule or mass suspected of malignancy, signs of active tuberculosis, sequelae of tuberculosis, bronchiectasis, signs of pneumonia.
- Associated signs

2- Vascular study:

- Pulmonary systemic circulation :
    - Signs pointing to the bleeding artery :
    - Pathological ASB detected: number, origin of each (orthotopic or ectopic), diameter at the carina, degree of tortuosity and traceability.
    - Pathological ASNB detected: number, origin and route.

    - Presence of dangerous anastomoses: an anterior spinal artery.

- Pulmonary arterial circulation :
    - Pulmonary embolism.
    - Pulmonary artery aneurysm.
    - Arterio-bronchial fistula.

CONCLUSION :

Most likely cause of bleeding

Stigmata of recent bleeding localised to ... or diffuse, with an estimated extent of ....

Systemic bronchial and/or non-bronchial hypervascularisation of the lobe/lung ...

No pulmonary artery anomaly.

MASSIVE HEMOPTYSIS: ROLE OF MULTIDETECTOR COMPUTED TOMOGRAPHY BEFORE BRONCHIAL ARTERY EMBOLIZATION

Abstract

Introduction:

Massive hemoptysis is rare yet life-threatening due to the risk of asphyxia. The role of multi-detector computed tomography (MDCT) in its handling has yet to be defined. The objectives of our study were to describe the role of MDCT in determining the site of bleeding in massive hemoptysis by comparing its data with that of conventional angiography (CA) and to look for predictive radiological criteria of bleeding recurrence after bronchial artery embolization (BAE).

Methods:

This was a descriptive study including clinical and radiological records of 58 patients, admitted, between June 2008 and November 2021, to pneumology department of Mohamed Taher Maamouri or Sahloul hospital for massive hemoptysis. They underwent MDCT in the radiology department of the same hospital and were treated by BAE in Sahloul hospital.

Results:

MDCT found parenchymal bleeding stigmatain 79,3% cases, localized in one pulmonary lobe in 60,4% of the cases. We found no difference between predominant site of bleeding signs at MDCT and the culprit bronchial artery on CA ($p>0,005$). The most frequent etiology of bleeding was bronchial dilatation (37.9%). Matching results between MDCT and CA were obtained in 91,3% in the depiction of culprit bronchial systemic arteries (BSA) and 80% in non-bronchial systemic arteries (NBSA). MDCT had a sensitivity of 80% and specificity of 62,5% in the depiction of culprit BSA and 80% and 84,6% in the depiction of culprit NBSA. MDCT was more sensitive in the depiction of culprit NBSA. Immediate bleeding control was achieved in 93,1% of the cases. Rebleeding rate was 51,7%. Rebleeding was significantly more frequent when bleeding signsextent exceeded 50% of pulmonary parenchyma ($p=0,003$). Rebleeding risk was significantly higher when NBSA (OR=1,6) or pulmonary circulation were implicated (OR=1,9 and OR=2). All cases of aspergilloma experienced rebleeding.

Conclusion:

MDCT plays a crucial role in massive hemoptysis management. It is sensitive and specific in the localization of bleeding site and the depiction of culprit artery to guide its catheterization during BAE. It can also predict rebleeding risk.

Keywords: Massive hemoptysis, Computed tomography angiogram, Angiography, Balloonembolization, Prognosis

MASSIVE HEMOPTYSIS: THE ROLE OF ANGIOSCANNING PRIOR TO BRONCHIAL EMBOLISATION

Summary

Introduction :

Massive haemoptysis is rare, but can be life-threatening due to the risk of asphyxia. The role of thoracic CT angiography in its management remains to be defined. The aims of our study were to describe the role of thoracic CT angiography in determining the site of bleeding by comparing its data with that of conventional pre-embolisation angiography, and to identify radiological severity criteria predictive of recurrence.

Methods :

Descriptive study of 58 radio-clinical records of patients admitted, between June 2008 and November 2021, to the Pneumology Department of Mohamed Taher Maâmouri Hospital in Nabeul or Sahloul Hospital for massive haemoptysis, explored by a DTA in the Medical Imaging Department of the same hospital and treated by embolisation at Sahloul Hospital.

Results :

CT angiography revealed signs of recent bleeding in 79.3% of cases, localised bleeding in 60.4% of cases. There was no difference between the site of predominance of parenchymal signs of bleeding on CT scan and the side of the culprit artery on angiography ($p>0.005$). The most common cause of bleeding was bronchiectasis (37.9%). Concordance between CT and angiography in the detection of culprit bronchial systemic arteries (BSA) and non-bronchial systemic arteries (NBSA) was 91.3% and 80% respectively. TDCT had a sensitivity of 84% and a specificity of 62.5% for the detection of culprit ASBs and 80% and 84.6% for the detection of culprit ASNBs, respectively. ATDM was more sensitive than angiography in detecting ASNB. Immediate control of bleeding after embolisation was achieved in 93.1% of cases. The recurrence rate was 51.7%. Recurrence was significantly more frequent in the case of bleeding stigmata extending to more than 50% of the lung parenchyma ($p=0.003$). The risk of recurrence was significantly greater in cases involving an ASNB (OR=1.6) and the pulmonary arterial circulation in the bleeding (OR=1.9 and OR=2). All cases of aspergilloma recurred.

Conclusion:

DTA plays a vital role in the management of massive haemoptysis. It is sensitive and specific in locating the artery responsible for the bleeding, to guide catheterisation during embolisation. It can also be used to predict recurrence of bleeding.

Key words: Massive haemoptysis, Angioscan, Angiography, Balloon catheter embolisation, Prognosis

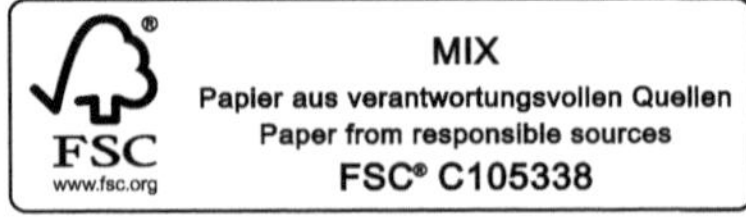

Printed by Books on Demand GmbH, Norderstedt / Germany